The Ultimate Guide
to Sexual Fantasy

Ultimate Guides from Cleis Press

The Ultimate Guide to Adult Videos
by Violet Blue

The Ultimate Guide to Anal Sex for Men
by Bill Brent

The Ultimate Guide to Anal Sex for Women
by Tristan Taormino

The Ultimate Guide to Cunnilingus
by Violet Blue

The Ultimate Guide to Fellatio
by Violet Blue

The Ultimate Guide to Pregnancy for Lesbians
by Rachel Pepper

The Ultimate Guide to Sex and Disability
by Miriam Kaufman, MD, Cory Silverberg and Fran Odette

The Ultimate Guide to Strap-On Sex
by Karlyn Lotney

The Ultimate Guide to Sexual Fantasy

How to Turn Your
Fantasies into Reality

VIOLET BLUE

CLEIS
PRESS

Published in the United States by Cleis Press Inc.,
P.O. Box 14684, San Francisco, California 94114.

Printed in the United States.
Cover design: Scott Idleman
Cover photograph: Doralba Picerno
Text design: Karen Quigg
Cleis Press logo art: Juana Alicia
First Edition.
10 9 8 7 6 5

LIBRARY OF CONGRESS CATALOGING-IN-PUBLICATION DATA

Blue, Violet.
    The ultimate guide to sexual fantasy : how to turn your fantasies into reality / by Violet Blue.— 1st ed.
        p. cm.
Includes bibliographical references and index.
    ISBN 1-57344-190-2 (pbk. : alk. paper)
    1. Sex instruction. I. Title.
    HQ56.B617 2004
    306.77—dc22
                                2004012792

Acknowledgments

Thanks especially to Felice Newman and Frédérique Delacoste—
my dear friends, staunch supporters, and real-life heroes at Cleis
Press.

Thomas Roche, thank you for being a true friend and wonderful
co-conspirator in the world of sex writing. Alison Tyler, with your
loving and wickedly dirty keystrokes, this book quivers with excitement—thank you for the hard work you did to make the stories a
"perfect fit." Carol Queen and Charlie Glickman, fellow sex edu-
cators, thank you! Special thanks to the many professionals I interviewed, who on occasion served my lover and myself as customers
for research purposes. Extra special thanks to Mistress Morgana,
escort Rose, and professional erotic masseuse Elizabeth R. Mandi:
you are my fetish muse. Thank-yous by the hundreds go out to
those who answered my ads and surveys, and joined my online
clubs and discussion groups. Thanks to the adventurous couples
who let me interview you—your relationships are inspiring.

Imagine being able to try out everything in this book with
someone you passionately love and feverishly lust after. For me
that person is my boyfriend, Courtney. "Thanks" doesn't convey
the ecstatic joy and pleasure I feel remembering our adventures
doing "research," and the thrill at imagining what's still to come.
Thank you for joining me on this wild, gleefully happy ride. Uz
jzme doma, my love.

Contents

Introduction:
The Mirror of Desire

Sexual fantasy is one of our great cultural obsessions—it is the mirror of desire, reflecting our own, and our lovers', faces. Books devoted to fantasies fly off the shelves of bookstores, encouraging our hunger for more. More fantasy, variety, something different; more unusual, bizarre, and titillating sexual daydreams; more ideas for shared sex play. We want our sex lives to be exciting and diverse, and we want to be electrified, shocked, intrigued, and stimulated by new and unusual ideas for sex.

The Ultimate Guide to Sexual Fantasy is for the thousands and thousands of women and men who want their sex lives to be an ever-changing menu of intimate daily specials. We all dream of making our fantasies come true—or at least making them vivid and heart-stopping, like a sexual thrill ride. Few of us tire of wanting to know our lovers' fantasies, and we continually quest to satisfy them.

I know this is true—because I've spoken to an endless stream of customers who visit the women-run sex toy store where I work. They want to know how to make coupled sex hotter and seek practical inspiration for spicing up their routine. It seems like everyone wants something hotter, newer, more arousing, more inspiring.

Up until recently, the problem was, we'd all read those old books of sexual fantasies, you know, those "tell-all" collections of "private therapy sessions" (yeah, right) and stories with tiresome moralistic or negative endings. Those books never were really supportive of threesomes, bisexuality, fetishes, or any but the most tame role-playing scenario.

With the intention of avoiding the moralistic, dated style of heterosexual fantasy books and tapping into the high quality and adventurousness typically found in more current erotica, I edited *Sweet Life: Erotic Fantasies for Couples* and *Taboo: Forbidden Fantasies for Couples*. I wanted to give these adventurous, loving couples— and singles—more to take to bed, so to speak. Every single fantasy in those books could realistically be replicated at home—or in the car, under the desk, at the restaurant…. *The Ultimate Guide to Sexual Fantasy* provides the "how-to" part of that equation. This guide explains how to make any sexual fantasy you can imagine come true. Here you'll find a huge wealth of practical ideas and real advice about sexual fetishes and fantasies. You'll find step-by-step instruction in fantasy negotiation and planning, role-playing, lap-dancing, stripping, S/M techniques, and more. You'll find examples of hundreds of fantasy roles and characters, and a complete guide to resources to help you find costumes, accessories, props, and toys. There's advice for introducing new ideas—no matter how silly or small, or profound and life-changing—into your shared sex life, as well as advice for coping with difficult or troubling fantasies.

With this guide, you will find out how to incorporate new sex acts, positions, sex in public, or edgy encounters—safely and pleasurably. Learn how to enjoy anal sex, deep throat, orgasms from penetration, or change the way you come, all by blending fantasy with your regular masturbation routines. Keep fantasies in your bedroom but make them authentic and realistic with the right details, props, and clothing. Take your fantasies out into the world: Have a threesome, an orgy, go to a sex party, try swinging, go to a strip club, visit a call girl or prostitute, or a dominatrix. Make your own porn, take erotic photos, or use the Internet in dozens of delightfully devious ways.

Here, you'll read how role-play can be fun, and hot, and not as goofy to try as you may think. If you already enjoy role-play you can take it to the limits of ecstasy. Overcome shyness and learn to talk dirty, strip, perform a lap dance, give your lover phone sex, or an erotic massage. If S/M and kinky play sound exciting, learn all the things you can do with BDSM in a kinky context, and for once, walk away from a book with concrete ideas about what to do as a dominant, submissive, or captive; what to do with someone all tied up—or simply how to ask for a spanking. Do you or does your lover have a fetish for feet, panties, uniforms, rubber—or something more exotic? Learn how to make fetish and sex work together to become a sex toy hotter and more reliable than one anything you can buy in a store. And there is a huge resource list in Chapter 13 to keep you moving, get you going, experimenting, and finding the things that turn you on the most.

The Ultimate Guide to Sexual Fantasy is a warm welcome to the world of fantasy fulfillment. May you—and your partners—continue changing and loving and experimenting, and may all your erotic dreams comes true.

Violet Blue
San Francisco
July 2004

Choose Your Own Adventure

Have you ever wondered what it would be like to go to a sex party? Thought about a threesome? Imagined tying up your lover for an evening of erotic power—or submission? Perhaps you've always wanted to pretend you were schoolgirl, or a doctor. Or in your own private moments, perhaps you dream of being seduced by a rock star. Or your partner has confessed to a fantasy of being a sexy firefighter saving pretty girls from danger. Have you ever thought about doing the most forbidden sex act you could think of with that new secretary, in the office, after hours?

Think of sexual fantasy as the cornerstone of your individual sexual expression. An erotic fantasy is any thought, idea, image, or scenario that interests you sexually. It doesn't necessarily have to turn you on, or by contrast it can be the one thing that gets your blood boiling.

If you think you don't fantasize, think again. Fantasies emerge from your erotic imagination in countless different forms, from fragmented sexual snippets to incredibly detailed narratives. Imagining romance, dreaming of someone you find attractive, masturbating to stories of taboo or even impossible sex, and vividly conjuring scenarios or sexual couplings you hope to make real in the near future are all ways we experience sexual fantasy.

Why do people like to fantasize about sex so much? Ever tried an aphrodisiac that worked? Not many people have. Even the legendary "Spanish Fly" is a myth—but sexual fantasies truly are Mother Nature's 100 percent natural, guaranteed aphrodisiac.

Fantasy can make masturbation intense and focused. You can set aside an hour just for your own pleasure, and include lubricant, a reliable toy such as a vibrator, and a fantasy—conjured by your own imagination, or taken from pictures in a book or magazine, or an adult movie.

Fantasy helps us to feel sexually self-reliant. Masturbating to a reliable fantasy and enjoying how good you can make yourself feel is one of the most empowering things you can do.

Try casting yourself in the starring role of your favorite X-rated film, whether in your head while masturbating, while watching the action onscreen, or in real life, with a lover.

Or get out of a sexual rut, no matter if you're single or in a couple, by finding new fantasies to explore. For ideas, read erotica and sex-tip books such as this one, explore the wide world of porn or romance movies, or visit Internet chat rooms as a voyeur.

You can "try on" sexual activities in fantasy. Think of it as an imaginary dress rehearsal. What would it be like to fellate your well-endowed new boyfriend or spank your new girlfriend's ample bottom?

You can go to extremes without real-life risks; in fact, you can vividly imagine any far-out sexual scenario that turns you on, without risking a thing. You can role-play scenarios that would be dangerous or taboo in real life, such as sex with a stranger, with many strangers, kidnapping, age play, forced sex, and more.

Spice up your shared sex life and reach deeper levels of intimacy with your partner by sharing tried-and-true fantasies and discovering new ones. You can build up to trying out your favorite fantasies in real life.

With fantasy, you can enjoy sexual activities and scenarios you're not experiencing on your own or in your relationship. Sometimes we want something our partners don't. Fantasy portrayals, watching what you want in porn, and well-planned masturbation sessions can get you what you want without upsetting your relationship.

Sometimes when we tell others what we like to fantasize about, our scenarios become others' fantasies as well. And when we brag to friends about real-life exploits, we never know which stories, innocently told over morning coffee, will become that evening's erotic fodder—or the script for your best friend's weekend tryst. We can make our fantasies real, if we choose—or in some cases, if we dare. You'll read more on this topic throughout the book.

Fantasies are your own private, personal sex toys. They send a direct current buzzing from your brain down to your groin. The right sexual fantasy, running in your head like your own private movie, can turn you on like a switch. When you know what works for you, your own vivid imagination can bring you to dizzying heights of arousal—and take you over the orgasmic edge.

Fantasy and Fetish

While fantasies tend to appear as scenarios—elaborate or simple—fetishes involve the erotic objectification of very specific items, symbols, or actions. Often the fetishized object of desire is something that might not be thought of as sexual or even erotic by someone who doesn't share the fetish.

Fetishes are typically viewed as something for those with far-out tastes—people in the bizarre end of the sexual gene pool—or as something reserved for sexual mavericks. However, because fetishes are target-specific arousal triggers, many people have a sexual fetish of some kind, whether mild or wild. Someone might fetishize certain uniforms or shoes, overlarge cocks or breasts, rubber isolation suits, or even women smoking cigarettes. And while one person may occasionally like his lover to wear a nurse's uniform, another absolutely can't get off unless there are pastries present or balloons being crushed. You can reassure yourself that having a fetish is a normal, healthy expression of self-defined sexuality.

Since fetishes are so specific, they are easy to incorporate into fantasy play. You can read more about fetishes in Chapter 9, "Fetishes."

Popular Fantasy Themes

Get your fantasy-making machinery in motion by identifying some general themes that turn you on. Do you know what turns you on? What shape do your fantasies take? Are they vivid, vague, seemingly mundane, or a little scary? Don't try to look deeply into their meanings just yet; instead, pick out the main themes. What you're doing is isolating what makes your favorite fantasy a peak erotic experience for you. Keep your mind open, and don't pass judgment on yourself—this isn't about "good" and "bad," it's about understanding what turns you on. Note the important differences between what is possible in fantasy and what is possible in reality. Here are some popular erotic themes:

Being Restrained
Held down, tied up, mummified, handcuffs, rope, bondage, tied to a chair, tied to the bed, tied to another person or yourself, rendered physically helpless in some way, caged, on a collar and leash, sensory restraint such as a blindfold or gag, held down by another person.

Being "Used"
A slave, a fuck toy, being limp or lifeless, getting passed around by multiple partners, your mouth or genitals used for someone else's gratification, face-sitting, gloryholes, the football team.

Casual or Anonymous Partners
A stranger in a bar, sex with anyone you don't know, with the waitress, with the UPS guy, as a sex worker or a porn star, while masked, as a burglar, a stranger in an adult movie theater, sex party, or bathhouse.

Fetishes
Feet, breasts, butts, dicks, mouths, panties, high heels, boots, overly large body parts, inflation, rubber and leather clothing, urine, feces, smoking, balloons being

squished or popped, pastries, pony play, knives, a particularly meaningful article of clothing, uniforms, Catholic schoolgirl attire, Santa Claus, long hair, pubic hair (or lack of), virgins, fat folks.

Firsts

First time doing vaginal intercourse, oral sex, anal sex, first time as a sex worker, first sexual experimentation, such as with a babysitter, an older sexual teacher, a younger student.

Gender Play

Dressing in drag, strapping it on, a woman having sex as a man, a man having sex as a woman, discovering (or knowing) that "she" is a "he," a preference for transsexual sex partners, androgynous sex partners, people with male and female genitalia, sissy boys and sissy maids.

Being in Control

Exerting sexual power, having people "service" you, being an S/M top, owning a sexual slave, forcing your lover to do your sexual bidding, using your partner as a sex toy, erotic dominance, sexual initiation ("taking the virgin"), tying up your lover, making sexual rules, shaving your partner, dressing her in a collar or panties, leading the sexual action, ganging up on your lover with others, erotically spanking someone naughty.

Loss of Control

Someone has sexual power over you and makes you do things, being helpless, powerless, in the hands of a robber or a cop, tied up or spanked, being the submissive or bottom, letting your lover call the shots and lead the action, being instructed on how to dress or behave in an erotic context, being "pimped out" or exhibited, being unable to control your sexual urges. (See Being "Used," above).

Multiple Partners

A gang bang (one person with four or more partners), sex with a sports team or a rock band, sex party, orgy, "ganging up" on your lover with friends, a threesome (two girls and one guy—or two guys and one girl), being arrested by a squad of cops, being used and abused by cheerleaders, enlisting your lover's help in seducing the girl or boy at the café (or picking up a male or female sex worker), sex with another couple, with a stripper in a club.

Public Spaces

At the office (at work), in a bar, bathroom, movie theater, park, department-store dressing room, alleyway, elevator, parked car, restaurant, subway or train, bus, parking lot or garage, on a rooftop, beach, street corner, onstage, behind the counter, at a sex club or private party, a strip club, in front of strangers—or friends.

Role Play

You (or your partner) are an icon: a cop or highway patrol officer, robber, schoolgirl, hooker, stripper, porn star, doctor, nurse, teacher, human animal such as a pony or dog, human animal owner or trainer, cheerleader, football team captain, babysitter, beach bunny, leatherman, age play (when one is older or younger), sci-fi creatures, aliens, a pimp, delivery person, plumber, traveling sales person, attacker, victim, salesgirl, waiter or waitress, bellhop.

Romance

Dreamy settings and seductions: being seduced by a rock star or actor, making love tenderly to the girl at the office, being rescued by a hot and horny fireman, saving your sexy fantasy lover from danger, a surprise fantasy enactment, seduction by candlelight, a sexy bath together, a dreamy getaway, sex in an exotic setting, a sexy picnic, perhaps with food on your lover's body, stripping or lap dancing for your lover, being sexually irresistible.

Taboo

With a forbidden person like clergy or family, with an animal, same gender, significant age difference, inappropriate urges or timing, rape, nonconsensual sex, in dangerous settings, abduction, knives, blood play, gang bangs, being "used" or experiencing a loss of control (see above) urination, defecation, enemas, necrophilia, gender play (see above).

Voyeurism

Watching people have sex, through the bushes or from outside their house, secretly watching a man or woman undress or masturbate, watching people have sex on TV, seeing another person (like a single woman) watch sex acts, a sex party, watching a sex worker, openly watching a masturbator, watching porn, watching a sex show or peep show, hidden cameras.

Your Current or Past Partner

A memory of a real-life event, imagining a fantasy you hope to do together, imagining your partner behaving differently than usual—such as being dominant or submissive, thinking of what you'd like to do to your lover, fantasizing about an old lover, thinking about your present partner having sex with your ex (or all three of you together).

When Fantasies Make You Feel Bad

Often we fantasize about scenarios that should never happen (or that we *wish* had never happened)—and some that aren't even possible. We may fantasize about humiliating others or exerting control over them—and not in the context of a consensual scene. We may fantasize about our own experiences of sexual abuse. We may be ashamed to admit what fantasies we entertain.

Fantasies and fetishes are so culturally misunderstood, we may not even understand our own turn-ons. This can make us feel "bad" for enjoying them, leading us to become sexually isolated. Exploring your fantasies might upset you, even turn you off so powerfully you have to wonder what *that* was all about.

Some people don't care to explore their fantasies. Because fantasies arise in our imagination and therefore are connected to our subconscious, they can be startling, unpredictable, and sometimes even shocking. When we become aroused it's easy to surrender ourselves to whatever movie we're running in our heads—but sometimes, afterward, we realize that what got us off went beyond what we deem acceptable in our daily lives. It's easy to feel guilt or shame after a fantasy about a sexual act we find unpleasant or offensive. This can make us feel bad about sex, our desires, even who we are.

If the fantasy is powerful and includes something that in real life would cause us to feel shame or remorse, like degrading ourselves or betraying a loved one, it's easy to become upset. When fantasies involve the people who share our lives (as they are bound to do), they can make us very uncomfortable.

Sometimes it's not the content of the fantasies that triggers guilt, but rather when or where the fantasy occurs. Fantasies can happen at inconvenient or inappropriate times, such as at work or at the doctor's office, creating a sexually charged mood while the world innocently goes on around us. This may feel "dirty." Or you might find yourself fantasizing during sex with a partner: Your partner is fully present, yet unaware that you are imagining all sorts of things, even acts with other people, to get yourself off. The illusion is created that somehow you've betrayed your lover. It's important to understand the role of sexual fantasy in sex before beating yourself up about what, how, with whom, or when you fantasize.

We all know that fantasy is not reality. But when we masturbate and imagine troubling things, people, or situations, human curiosity kicks in and we ask ourselves whether these things are what we really want. For some people this is a horrifying thought. It's important to keep in mind that the realm of fantasy is a sanctuary in your mind where you are free to enjoy things that you would never do in real life.

Real-life relationships and your sexual fantasies (no matter how troubling) can work together beautifully once you understand what fantasies are, and how to use them. We can't help but indulge in certain fantasies, such as nonconsensual sex, age-inappropriate sex, or infidelity, nor can many of us resist getting aroused by them. And because we want our relationships to include every little thing that gets us hard or wet, our perceived lack of control over the acceptable boundaries of our fantasies can make us feel like we've stumbled into a danger zone It's as if what is safe is at odds with what is arousing. The two notions don't have to be at odds, and the act of bringing them together is a conscious one.

Fantasy Research

Fantasy source material can come from a variety of places. Obviously, there's your own imagination, but for some, hot ideas spring first from real-life sexual experiences. Real-life experiences can provide endless erotic inspiration, yet for many people what really gets the juices flowing (pardon the pun) is experiences we only wish we'd had. What if you *had* gone home with that stranger? Or *really* tried to get out of that speeding ticket?

Other ideas come from movies, music videos, porn, TV shows, books, and of course, erotica. And if you're not single, some of the steamiest ideas will come from your lover.

Remember that if you fantasize about something shocking, like being forced to perform sex, it doesn't mean that you want it to happen or that you are a bad person. But by identifying your fantasy scenario, you can find a safe space where imagination fuels desire.

By learning how to turn yourself on with fantasy, you can do extraordinary things, like make yourself really aroused and teach yourself new masturbation techniques. Or you can fantasize while your partner goes down on you, and learn to orgasm from the combination of oral stimulation *plus* fantasy. If you have established trust and sexual communication with a partner, you can share your fantasies—you can even make some of them come true. And in the following chapters, I'll tell you exactly how.

The Perfect Match

BY ALISON TYLER

After several months of dating, Miles and I were completely comfortable together. "The perfect match," I told my best friend. "Really and truly perfect." I felt okay stripping down in front of him, had gotten over the new-lover jitters, found that I slept better when he was next to me in bed, his strong arms curled around my body. I no longer needed my own space. But I suppose I shouldn't have felt so at ease so quickly. Letting down your guard can be dangerous. I've learned from the past, yet still, I found myself relaxing.

That's when he asked me to tell him my number one fantasy, and the thing was, I liked him. *Really* liked him. This wasn't a fling. It was real. So I did what any other girl would do in my situation—I lied. We'd only been together a short while, and I didn't want to scare him off. I've been in that situation before, cuddled up against a new man, sharing the sort of sexy secrets that make me the wettest, feeling faux safety while nuzzling against a barrel-chested lover. And then hearing the shock in his voice: "You want *what?*" and knowing it was all over.

This time, I was in it for the long haul. I adored Miles. If he didn't want to play dirty, then that was okay. I'd get my kink solo style, touching myself and envisioning all the twisted ways I like to get off. I'd save those seductive fantasies for myself, and get the rest of my needs fulfilled by my man.

But this man wasn't letting me get off so easy. "Come on, kiddo," he insisted. "What rocks your world? What do you like the best?"

"Oh, you know, what every girl likes."

"All girls are different."

"Well, then, whatever *you* like."

"That's just not true." He pushed up on one arm and looked at me. "Don't you trust me, Lia? Can't you tell me?"

I shrugged and said, "Sometimes."

"No time like the present," he countered.

"Later," I promised. "You tell me first."

"Fair enough," he said, curling back up with me again. "I've got this fantasy that I've been wanting to share with you—"

I could feel him getting hard again, and I pushed back against him so that we were pressed tight together.

"I want to spank that lovely ass of yours until you confess your favorite fantasy to me. Does that sound like something that would work for you?"

The muffled sigh that escaped me told him that he'd struck a chord, and within a second I found myself over his lap, ass in the air, his firm, steady hand connecting rapidly with my blushing backside. Maybe this man *would* be the one to hear out my dirty secrets, I thought, twisting in his embrace to find that I was unable to get free. That made me even wetter. When on the receiving end of a spanking, I don't want to be able to get free. I want to be held in place and forced to take my punishment. Who'd have thought that my handsome new boyfriend would understand this so quickly?

"Tell—" he insisted, reminding me of our game. "Tell now or you won't be able to sit down for a week."

I didn't want to sit down for a week.

"Tell," he said, "or I'll get my belt."

Oooh, a belt!

But finally, as the blows rained down faster and harder, I started talking, feeling more safe and secure than I ever had before. Here was a man who knew I needed a spanking. He just knew it. Without me having to explain. Without me needing to drop hints, to wear short schoolgirl skirts, to be bratty and naughty and tease him until he couldn't stand it. So maybe he'd be able to give me the rest of the things I needed as well.

"It starts like this," I said, and he pressed his hand against my hot skin and listened while I spoke. He didn't take me off his lap, though. He forced me to confess my fantasies while remaining in the awkward position of a recently punished plaything.

"You put me over your lap," I said.

"Yeah?" I could hear the smile in his voice.

"You put me over your lap and you take down my panties and let them dangle from my ankles. You set your firm, hard hand against my naked skin and let me guess how much it's going to hurt before you even start.

"How much is it going to hurt?" he asked.

"Oh," I sighed. "A lot. A good spanking has to really hurt."

"And then—"

"And then you spank my ass until it's all pretty and pinky-red, and while you spank me, you tell me what a naughty girl I am...."

"You are a naughty girl, you know," he said.

"Yeah, I know."

"But there's more, isn't there?"

"Of course," I said, thinking to myself: *Of course there's more. There's always more.* "You spank me until I squirm against you, but you don't let me go. And when you're finished—not me, but you—then you take me over to the mirror and let me see my hot, blushing bottom reflected back at me."

"Like this?" Miles asked, lifting me off his lap and pulling me quickly to the bedroom mirror. I gazed at my reflection over my shoulder, and then I met his eyes in the mirror, and I nodded. Yeah, like that. Just like that.

I guess we really are a perfect match.

Fantasies for One

Whether you want to make your fantasies come true, invent new fantasy scenarios, make your masturbation sessions hotter, or find peace of mind by understanding your fantasies, there's only one place to start: yourself. Fantasy, and how you like to use it, comes from inside you.

Masturbation: Just Do It

Everyone masturbates, and while our feelings about it range from shame to pride, and our masturbatory sessions from mechanical to joyous, we all have one thing in common: Each of us has a fantasy image or scenario playing out somewhere in our heads while we get off.

Volumes have been written about the health benefits of masturbation, refuting the harmful myths that have kept people from feeling good about engaging in this natural, normal activity. For some people, masturbation is a moment of release, something they'd prefer to get over with as soon as possible. For others, masturbation is regarded fondly, as something healing, rewarding, relished in whatever form it takes. When we masturbate, we are doing something nice for ourselves, bringing oxygen and blood to our genitals, exercising our pelvic muscles, and keeping them healthy and strong. We're also getting off, plain and simple—and it feels damn good.

Masturbation is where it all begins for us sexually, from our earliest orgasms to our first discoveries of how we like to be touched. For all of our sexual experiences, this is the place where we can return for reference and new information, a sexual dictionary of our own unique terms. When we want to try something new, such as adult videos, vibrators, or even a new sex technique with a partner, masturbation is the best tool we've got to help get us started.

Fantasy fuels our masturbation sessions. Even when our arousal is purely physiological, a hot fantasy can aid a skilled hand. Arousal, masturbation, and fantasy combined can be a powerful tool for learning how to:

- Orgasm better, harder, faster, more reliably.
- Orgasm during sex acts such as giving or receiving oral sex, anal sex, intercourse.
- Overcome sexual fear or anxiety; for example, sex with a new partner, arousal difficulties from stress, nervousness when trying new things.
- Change sexual habits; for example, trying new sensations such as anal sex or light pain (S/M), learning to masturbate to new stimulus, increasing or decreasing frequency.

Hot Masturbation Sessions: Fantasies, Sex Toys, and More

So, you've got your favorite fantasies, and you love to masturbate thinking about them—how can you make them more real? Easy: a little forethought, and maybe a shopping trip or two.

Public masturbation fantasies are tricky, but not impossible. Be very aware of the laws about public sex in your area. If you get caught, you will likely go to jail—or at least get booked and arraigned—not as sexy in real life as in fantasy, I assure you. Make absolutely sure that no one will see you. It's part of the thrill, the threat of discovery, but if someone sees you, you are involving him or her in a sex act without his or her consent—this is not okay. Seek out reliably secluded spots, such as a remote place to park, a deserted natural area like a beach or forest, a vacant warehouse, an empty movie theater.

Some places in large cities are notorious for being public sex spots—use these places only if you are a local and are familiar with the area. If you must cruise, proceed with streetwise caution. Rooftops can seem public but still be private. Look around first, before you're horny. Think ahead about places to duck for cover, ways to camouflage your activity, or a story to tell an authority figure. Make it as hot and fun as you can—public masturbation is a thrilling encounter that can never be exactly duplicated. Don't hold back. Read about safety and good locations in Chapter 8, "Public Sex."

Explicit visuals can bring your fantasies into your living room in living color. Adult videos and images in porn books and magazines can depict precisely the acts that make you horny. You can allow yourself to mentally sink into the scene as you masturbate to orgasm. You "become" the woman with the penis in her mouth; you "become" the man penetrating her.

Mirrors take erotic imagery to the next level for those already comfortable with watching explicit sex, and can be a terrific education for those who have never seen themselves up close—or while sexually stimulated. You don't necessarily need porn to make your fantasy more visceral—some may even find it distracting, or dislike the medium of porn. The best imagery is always going to be in your head, anyway! With a well-positioned mirror, you can provide your own visuals by watching your genitals, or entire body, as you masturbate. A small mirror can be propped up in your bed or on the floor, or you can sit in front of a full-length mirror and experiment with watching yourself in different positions. Taking your time to drizzle and massage lube on yourself is twice as hot when you can see every move your hands make—and don't be afraid to talk dirty!

Sex toys are not only excellent masturbation tools—they also make wonderful props for your fantasy scenarios. Sex-act-specific fantasies—anal sex, oral sex, penetration, S/M—can be simulated with a variety of sex toys and gear. Would a dildo in your mouth make that group-sex fantasy more real? Would a butt plug enhance the medical fantasy? A nipple clamp bring your dungeon to life?
　　Here are some deliciously naughty toys and ideas:

> **Dildos** are phallic-shaped, nonvibrating sex toys
> used for penetration, and they can be employed
> in a variety of fantasy scenarios. Someone being

"forced" to suck cock might drag a dildo all around their face, then force it into their own mouth repeatedly, something you can easily do with one hand while masturbating with the other. Any fellatio fantasy can be enhanced with a dildo, and imagining group sex is certainly more fun with multiple dildos. Gender play takes off when you wear a dildo in a harness, masturbating the dildo and yourself at the same time. Vibrating dildos add a buzz to the festivities. Dildo masturbation combined with fantasy is a great way to learn how to orgasm from penetration.

Anal toys add sensation to anal sex fantasies. Some people may simply enjoy stimulation from their own finger, or the "threat" of insertion

What Not to Stick in Your Butt

What if you don't have any anal toys handy at the crucial moment? No doubt you've heard urban legends about people going to the ER with all manner of odd and potentially lethal items lodged in their rectums—and unfortunately, quite a few of these stories are true. Don't make a hasty decision about toys for anal play. Make the right choice when you stimulate your ass: Even if you're ashamed or unwilling to admit what excites you, we're talking about avoiding embarrassment and serious injury. Always use lots of lubrication—the skin around the anus tears easily, but won't if it's well-lubed. Never put something in your butt—or anywhere near your butt—that has sharp edges, can possibly break, shatter, or crack, or doesn't have a significantly flared base for easy retrieval. Your lubed anal sphincter will pull in anything you put inside, and if you can't grab it safely to pull it back out, you're off to starring in your own urban legend. Carrots are right out—get the right tool for the job, such as a butt plug or a dildo safe for anal use.

from a finger or small plug, sending whatever anal-sex scenario is running in their heads into overdrive. Anal beads can be inserted one at a time, left in, or pulled out slowly or quickly, depending on the fantasy. Or you can go further, becoming a fantasy "anal queen" (or anal slut), using increasingly bigger and bigger butt plugs to stimulate yourself while imagining a multitude of anal slaves servicing you in your love sling. Larger toys, used safely, can exacerbate the feeling of "violation," and any penetration toy can be employed to enhance the fantasy of being taken by force, or being "used." Butt plugs can also be inserted and left in place during other activities, for a variety of fantasies such as submission, slavery, and medical scenarios—or just to free up your hands to get the dildo into your mouth.

Masturbation sleeves for men add a whole new dimension of sensation to the usual one- or two-handed action. These sleeves come in a variety of shapes, thicknesses, materials, and colors—choose the one you find most appealing. Some might find the tiny fake buttholes on some of these toys creepy, while others might find them erotically interesting. Would that enhance your fantasy of having anal sex with a porn star? Give it a try. If tit-fucking is your fantasy *du jour*, semirealistic molded breasts might give your next session an edge. Either way, these toys are harmless. Using them doesn't mean you want to have sex with a body part, or are somehow unable to have sex with the whole woman, they're just toys for healthy adult sex play. Explore and enjoy your fantasies to the fullest—at the very least, you'll experience a new sensation on your penis while your masturbate.

Sensation and S/M toys make your pleasure/pain fantasies much more real Be sure to use caution and common sense when you play alone with pain, bondage, electricity, asphyxiation, or any toy that induces strong sensations. Little clamps and clips can be used safely to intensify pinching sensations, though keep in mind that they hurt much more when you take them off, as the blood rushes back to the previously clamped area. These items can be purchased in a sex toy or S/M boutique, a hardware store, or a stationery store. Test them on the soft flesh of your arm before you buy—looks can be deceiving, and they can hurt worse than they look. Be sure that the ends of your clips are encased in rubber, and don't buy ones with teeth. Clips and clamps can be placed on the fleshy parts of the body: breasts, nipples, stomach, thighs, labia, skin of the penis and testicles, even lips and earlobes! Apply your clips according to your fantasy scenario, but don't leave them on for longer than your masturbation session.

Some S/M scenarios are difficult and dangerous to simulate. While you may be able to flog yourself, putting yourself into bondage (handcuffs, ropes, restraints, silk scarves, and so on) is not at all recommended. Asphyxiation, while not uncommon as a fantasy, is extremely dangerous to attempt, especially alone, and all too often can be fatal. Electrical play leaves much room for error—lethal error—and should be done only by those experienced with electricity, or learned from an expert in electricity and S/M. Blindfolds are fine, as long as you will be safe without being able to see.

Change Habits and Learn New Tricks

When you see a picture, watch a movie, read a story, or have an idea that really turns you on—as in: wet panties or stiffening cock—you've got a fantasy that works for you. You can learn to mine your masturbatory fantasies for arousal tools. Take a moment to recall your last masturbation session. What felt good? What were you thinking? Did you have a scenario in mind, a picture in your head? Were you watching a hot porn video? Don't worry about whether the idea or image is "good," "bad," or appropriate—right now you are simply using your erotic imagination as a tool. Think about how it started, the buildup, and what made you come. It's likely that you began with an idea; the images or action escalated in some way, then began to crescendo, and reached a peak that coincided with orgasm. Think about the beginning of your masturbation session, the start and the buildup—this is how you turn yourself on.

Digging into what turned you on most recently is a technique for becoming aroused again, and reliving the experience provides a stepping-stone to better controlling or intensifying your arousal. Get turned on, and try something new—allow yourself to become as aroused as you can stand, and see what images appear as you near orgasm.

To make your orgasms better, more intense, more reliable, and to explore multiple orgasms—including, for men, orgasm without ejaculation—take your time masturbating, and proceed as slowly as you can. Try taking yourself to the heights of arousal, but don't allow yourself to go over the edge—prolong the inevitable for as long as you can. Practitioners of Tantra use conscious breathing and slow sexual techniques to build up to intense orgasms. Men can learn to take themselves up to the edge of orgasm and, employing the "squeeze" technique, back off again, eventually learning how to have multiple orgasms, which means coming without ejaculation.

You can teach yourself new sexual techniques—and have a lot of fun in the process—using your newfound skill for conjuring up fantasies that turn you on. Having an orgasm during partnered sex, or from something you don't usually orgasm from, such as oral or anal sex, is possible when you employ arousal, masturbation, and

A Tool for Men: The Squeeze Technique

The squeeze technique is an easy way to keep yourself from coming before you or your partner is ready (and you don't need to use those potentially harmful—and questionably effective—"delay" creams or sprays). The squeeze is done by placing your hand at the tip of the penis so that the thumb is on the underside, or frenulum, with the fingertips placed on top, on the coronal ridge. When you get close, stop everything—especially any fantasies—and squeeze for three or four seconds. Some men find that squeezing at the base works best, and others find that pulling their balls down, away from the body, works just as well—experiment to see how you respond. To read more about orgasm techniques for men, pick up a copy of The Multi-Orgasmic Man, by Mantak Chia and Douglas Abrams.

fantasy techniques. It's a gradual process, but well worth the effort.

When you want to incorporate a new technique into your sex life, such as deep throating or vaginal fisting, begin by fantasizing about it when you masturbate. If you feel nervous or afraid, learn as much as you can about the new activity. Read about it, or watch an educational adult film—resources and recommendations can be found in Chapter 13, "Resources." On your own time, explore an angle that arouses your curiosity *(a whole hand would be hot)*—or that makes you hesitant *(doesn't it hurt?)*.

Fantasy is the most effective way to overcome masturbation habits you dislike or want to change, using similar techniques as above. Say, for instance, you usually orgasm quietly when you masturbate on your stomach—but want to learn to come loudly while on your back with your legs spread. Or you want to orgasm

A Tool for Women: Your Vibrator

Women who routinely use vibrators for masturbation take their trusty pal along on their fantasy explorations, but women who have never tried a vibe might also want to give it a whirl. Vibrators—or massagers—are excellent tools for exploring your arousal. Many women, even those who have had difficulty reaching orgasm, find that vibrators bring them easy arousal and reliable orgasms. Select a vibrator that looks appealing to you, and set aside time to enjoy your new toy free of distractions or possible interruptions. Start out by applying vibration to your inner thighs, slowly making your way up to your genitals. Experiment with speeds and pressure. After a few sessions of enjoyable exploration, add your vibrator to your solo fantasy adventures—and double your fun!

with penetration, or want to change a fetish such as masturbation with certain shoes. The shoes will always turn you on, but you can teach yourself to enjoy other activities sexually as well, mixing it up and making your sex life more dynamic.

Begin by becoming aroused in the ways most familiar to you, and use your reliable masturbation methods to bring yourself to the edge of orgasm. At this point, deliberately think about the aspects of the new behavior that turn you on the most—if it's anal sex, is it the new idea of anal stimulation itself, or perhaps that it's a "dirty" thing to do? Keep masturbating and fantasizing about the new activity, allowing yourself to orgasm with the hot fantasy—of you trying out the new behavior—running in your head as you come. Repeat the process until you feel ready to take your experimentation to the next level, which may take several masturbation sessions.

If you're feeling adventurous, couple your fantasy exercises with sex toys that can simulate sensation—such as a butt plug for anal intercourse, or a dildo for fellatio—or watch porn that graphically depicts the fantasy sex act you want to try.

The Golden Rules of Anal Masturbation

- Get yourself turned on before you attempt anal penetration.
- Go slowly. Very, very slowly.
- Use tons of lube.
- Tease yourself with massage or vibration on the outside first.
- Masturbate while you penetrate.
- Don't put anything dangerous in your ass.
- If it hurts, slow down, add lube, or switch activities.

Toys can help you explore anal sensation and help you define the line between comfort and pain. Playing with toys in masturbation gives your body a chance to trust the sensation while you're completely in control. Play with smooth, unbreakable toys that have a base so they can't slip inside, or insert fingers with trimmed nails, plus plenty of water-based lubricant. The tissue of the anus is thin, so nothing scratchy or sharp should be inserted.

Gradually you'll become more comfortable—and turned on—by the notion of trying out your fantasy in real life, and this can propel you toward some steamy encounters.

If you want to learn to deep-throat a penis using fantasy and masturbation, as with anal play, try it with a dildo as many times as you need to feel comfortable before doing it on a real, live person. Get a dildo with a flared end, so it is easy to hold on to—never use any-thing that could slip from your grasp, or break in your throat (no bananas or cucumbers). Practice breathing around the dildo and working around your gag reflex as you keep yourself turned on with masturbation and your hottest fantasies (preferably fantasies that include fellatio). Deep-throating, like anal sex, takes practice and patience.

To teach yourself to orgasm during partnered sex, or while giving or receiving oral sex, you can use the tech-niques above to get your arousal in step with your part-ner's. You don't have to fantasize about what you're doing while you're doing it—it helps to be turned on by the idea of what you're doing, but chances are this may not be your current number one fantasy. What's going to get you revved up and heading straight to orgasm is what turns you on most, so fantasize about what gets *you* hot. Use the fantasy that works for you, combined with the stimulation your lover is giving you, to come.

Some people are very uncomfortable with the idea of fantasizing during partnered sex. When you're having sex with your sweetie and your mind is somewhere else, it's easy to feel that you're being deceitful—though you're not, at all. You are right there with them, they are stimulating you, and you're fulfilling your part of the bargain perfectly by turning yourself on in the ways that work best for you so you can share your pleasure with them. You aren't doing anything wrong; in fact, you're doing what everyone else does when they have an orgasm, with or without a partner—using fantasy to kick-start your arousal, intensify the experience, and add variety to your sex life. A fantasy is simply something that works for you, be it a memory or an idea, and fantasizing during sexual activity is your way of incorporating it into your present relationship. Read more about fantasies for couples in the next chapter, "Fantasies for Two."

Three in One

BY ALISON TYLER

It happens so quickly that I don't know what to do. I have my hands inside my panties, touching myself in random, randy circles. Then suddenly, a second set of hands is on me, covering my eyes, and before I can fully react to that unexpectedly erotic development, yet another set of hands joins in, forcing my hands out of my satin bikini bottoms and touching my pussy for me.

I think it's a woman behind me and a man down below, only because of the softness of the hands covering my eyes and the roughness of those yanking my pretty pearly-white panties down my thighs and then spreading my pussylips wide apart. I feel how exposed I am, and I would blush if I had the time. But everything happens so quickly that I don't respond in any normal fashion. I don't scream. I don't fight. Not when the blindfold covers my eyes. Not when the feminine hands began to pinch my nipples, making them tent the slinky fabric of my semisheer T-shirt. I simply relax, relishing every second of the illicit experience. I groan as those rougher and ever-so-insistent hands on my sex stretch me wide and then wider, and I moan out loud when I feel a wet smear of lube drenching my inner lips.

"Oh, fuck me," I sigh, so wet, so very ready. "Please, fuck me—"

But though those hands are busy working me, nobody says a word. Fingers thrust forcefully into my pussy, and I clench down hard and lift my hips high in the air, savoring every second. I'm in heaven—the roughness of those hands palpitating my clit takes me on a delicious ride, alternating perfectly with the tightness of thumb and finger on my nipples pinching, harder, tighter. Hands caress me, rub over me, massage me.

"Oh, god," I sigh, and a large, hard cock finds my mouth. Now my moans and sighs are muffled by the rigid tool, but at least I have something to do, some sort of purpose. I start to suck on the cock, focusing on the way it feels, the way I instinctively know how to swallow it. I'm so overwhelmed by the pleasure of submitting that it takes me a moment before I realize a second cock is filling my pussy. Christ, so it was two men. One more feminine, perhaps, than the other. But that's okay. I'm ready. I can take them. I suck and suck, working the cock down my throat, and I can fuck and fuck, my pussy contracting on the cock inside me, bucking and thrusting, lost in this visionless world until…I feel a finger probing my asshole.

My body tenses. I'm scared at the intrusion, and I feel goose bumps rising on my skin. A chill flutters through me, shaking my entire body, but the finger is gentle, so gentle, and I sense the wetness of lube skating around my tender rear hole.

Around the cock in my mouth I form an excited O and rock back slowly, impaling myself on the probing digit.

Yes, I think. *Finger-fuck me there.* As if the unseen lover can read my mind, the finger obeys immediately, finger-fucking my asshole while my pussy is all stuffed full of cock. I'm going to explode, filled in three places, but I love every fucking second. The cock in my mouth thrusts deeper, faster, and I know I'm going to drain every drop. The hard member in my pussy works at a steadier rhythm, a deep thrust, in and out, then holds totally still while that finger goes into play again. But now, there's a second finger, pushing forward, overlapping, and I cry out around the cock in my mouth at how good that feels.

Oh, do I love a finger in my ass. Especially one so well-lubed and so slow to proceed. I'm going to come. I can sense it. I'm going to come in ribbons of pleasure, in waves of power. The invisible lover fucking my cunt understands this, and the cock pulls out and starts to gently fuck my clit, slipping back and forth in my ocean of wetness. I find that I'm on the verge of both creaming and screaming as that cock finds the rhythm I need. Now the owner of those venturing fingers in my ass starts to fuck me faster, working at a delicious pace.

I'm such a slut, I think, raising my thighs up in the air, holding them in place, spreading myself, my rear cheeks, so that the finger can drive in further. *Look,* I want to say. *Look at me here. See everything. I'm spreading myself. I'm revealing myself. Look at my asshole while you touch it.*

The cock in my mouth and the one at my clit fuck me together until I come, shuddering and sighing, nearly sobbing. And as soon as I start to come, the cock at my clit slides lower, and hands force me to roll onto my stomach. I turn my head carefully, still sucking the cock in my mouth, as the one behind me starts to press forward, butting against my rear hole. I shake my head forcibly, never relinquishing my hold on the cock I'm blowing, but I don't mean it—I don't mean "no." I want to come again. I'm a greedy little thing. I want to contract on that cock. I want to feel it in my asshole.

Slowly, so slowly, the cockhead teases its way in. I clench my eyes tight, and then the bulbous head is in me. I sigh with relief as the shaft slides easily forward.

Oh, yes. Oh, yes. I'm going to come again. This time with the cock in my asshole. I slide my own fingers under me to touch my clit while I'm getting a pounding in my rear hole. My fingers work faster; the cock thrusts harder, and then I'm there—at the finish, panting and sweating, and so high from the release that I let the cock slip from my mouth.

After a moment, I push the blindfold away, only to discover that I am alone in my bed. There are no strangers making love to me, only a few soiled dildos and a half-empty bottle of lube on the mattress at my side. I'm all by myself.

I grin when I think about tomorrow night. When I just might go for three in one once again.

Fantasies for Two

We are drawn to sexual indulgence, and we are engineered to share it with others. Seduction. Domination. Surprise. An outfit, setting, or prop that makes you irresistible and ignites passion. Watching your lover become aroused by your every move. Becoming his or her personal sex toy. Tasting something new that you've always wanted to try—with explosive results. When we feed each other the seductive treats of sexual fantasy, we find ourselves set for a wonderfully hedonistic erotic buffet.

When you and your lover uncork the magic bottle that holds your sexual fantasies, you might find yourselves swept from Kansas to Oz. From a fantasy whispered to each other during lovemaking all the way to a fully-costumed session of role-playing, sexual fantasies can make your ordinarily great sex life extraordinary.

Fantasies not only make your shared sex life sizzle—but they can also take the intimacy you already share to the next level, deepening lines of communication and strengthening your feelings for one another. Fantasies are full of excitement, thrill, danger, ecstasy, romance, and possibility. And they are perfect for sharing.

Building a Fantasy Scenario

Do you get turned on when you remember a particularly hot sexual position, perhaps with a twist or two, such as taking it public or with a sexy stranger watching? Although less elaborate than intricately staged role-playing—no costumes or particular shades of lipstick—the simplicity of fantasies based on remembered encounters belies their power to arouse.

Fantasy scenarios can take a premise like "secret hand job" and give it a context—like a movie theater, a restaurant, your desk at work, or an elevator. Take the fantasy further and the secret hand job in the movie theater comes from the stranger sitting next to you; in the restaurant it's from the waitress, and at the office it's from someone who really wants that job you're hiring for. And when you add costumes and props, clearly defined roles, a story line with a beginning, middle, and finish, you have smoothly transitioned to role-playing.

Basic fantasy scenarios come in limitless combinations, and I recommend using your intuition and your arousal as a barometer for determining what will work best for you—use your groin, not your brain. Combine fantasy elements that both turn you on and naturally seem to go together: a sex act, an item of clothing, and a place, a predicament.

You and your partner can participate equally—for example, doing sixty-nine in the back of a car. Or one of you may call the shots, running the show, with the other enjoying the ride (or being "forced" to go along with it).

Here are some suggestions to get you started. You can make your own list of fantasy elements that get you hot and bothered. Or copy the lists below; you and your partner can jot down "yes," "no," or "maybe" next to each item to get a clear idea of what you'd both like to play with.

Sex Acts

Masturbation, touching or masturbating through clothing, anal sex, rimming, oral sex, fisting, hand jobs, external ejaculation, ejaculation in mouth, female ejaculation, vaginal penetration, strap-on sex, threesomes, two couples, multiple partners, sex toys, male receptive anal penetration, female receptive anal penetration, particular positions such as doggie-style, being the middle of a "sandwich," face-sitting and "smothering," spanking, frottage (rubbing, as in a lap dance), sucking (nipples, clits, toes, cocks), licking (breasts, pussies, balls).

Clothing and Accessories

None (nude), panties, lingerie, men's clothing, neckties, boxer shorts, work clothes, shoes, boots, high heels, leather, lace, rubber, silk, bandages, collars, handcuffs, leashes, clothesline, glasses, ribbons, bows in hair, pigtails, barrettes, short skirts, formal dresses, tiaras, sentimental items like wedding garters, iconic items like letterman jackets, slippers, bathrobes, towels, aprons, strap-ons, sex toys such as vibrators or large dildos, gloves, lipstick, no makeup, long or short hair, hair color (brunettes or blondes), chairs, a couch, a bed.

Places and Predicaments

Household (kitchen, bedroom, closet, bathroom, toilet), cars, garage, motorcycle, fireplaces, barn or woodshed, beach, bars, alleyway, rooftop, caught in the act, punishment, "forced" sex, wrestling, competition, strangers, exhibitionism, in public, in a park, at work, a gas station, machine shop, dungeon, sex party, poolside, watching porn (especially a particular sex act), one nude while the other is clothed, locker rooms, embarrassment, control, fear, romance, seduction, sexy food play, restraint.

Did anything in these lists catch your attention? Spark a memory? Sound familiar? You can pick and choose which elements you'd like to make real and which might work better in the realm of imagination. Many couples would rather experiment with threesomes by pretending there is a third partner in the bed (employing their most inspired fantasy-fueled dirty talk) than by finding a real third partner to bring home. And it *is* much safer to send your husband to an imaginary dog house in your bedroom than to chain him up in the backyard. You can combine imaginary and real situations, people, and props in endless variations to get the most out of the fantasy scenarios that really turn you on.

In Your Head, or in Reality?

How "real" you make your fantasies is up to you. Generally speaking, you have many options when it comes to fantasy play within your relationship. You can:

• Keep your fantasies to yourself, enjoying them for masturbation or fantasizing during partnered sex.

- Share them by whispering your ideas or scenes to each other during sex.
- Confess a fantasy that you'd like to try—this will likely ignite some very hot sex—even if the fantasy remains in conversation.
- Talk openly about your fantasies together, and discuss ways in which you'd like to make them more realistic.
- Design the scenario in which you make your fantasies come true.

Successful fantasy play requires careful consideration of the circumstances, the timing, and your physical and emotional comfort. Most of all, it takes common sense. Let's face it, the idea of playing a sex worker who gets arrested by a gorgeous police officer—and is taken to the station for a sex-drenched afternoon in handcuffs—may sound appealing, but actually getting arrested isn't fun for anyone.

This is true for every fantasy you bring into reality, from playfully wearing panties under a business suit to forcing your boyfriend to have sex with a gang of bikers in a gas-station restroom. Consider all parameters of comfort and safety, and decide together how far you want to take the fantasy. The panties under his business suit may seem cute, but might compromise his behavior at the urinal—or make him go in the stall all day, causing him to feel more uncomfortable than sexy. Or feeling uncomfortable may be part of the fantasy: a subtle humiliation while you're not around to provide it yourself. He may not feel humiliation at all, just arousal, and you needn't worry—but you won't know unless you find out how far into the fantasy he'll stay sexually interested, and what limits will spoil the fun. Similarly, your partner may enjoy the idea of being "forced" into sex, but may react very negatively to being tied up, pushed around, or taken by surprise. Conversely, he may deeply desire all of these things, and despair that you don't go far enough.

How to Ask for a Spanking

One of my closest friends, a widely published erotica writer, surprised me with a confession when I told her about this book. She was excited to hear that there would be a resource for people who want to live their fantasies, and wished that it had been around for her when, almost ten years ago, she would've given almost anything to have her boyfriend spank her. "I always wanted to be spanked. But it took me two years to get my courage up and ask him—and he was mortified! I stayed with him for another year and I was miserable. When I asked my next boyfriend, he was upset too, because he thought that spanking was 'degrading' to women, and he'd never in a million years do that—but I told him that when she *wants* to be spanked, it's the opposite! About a week later he came over to my house with a hard-backed brush he bought, though he was still reluctant to use it, but I think that was mostly because he didn't know how."

All too often, we know what we want but don't know how to get it. You can muster your courage to ask for what you want, but that doesn't mean you'll be met with enthusiasm; or if you are, that your lover will have the information and skill to execute your desires in the ways you want. Opening up can be scary, and being met with shock, surprise, or distaste is even scarier. Learning how to discuss each other's desires, and picking up tips for starting the conversation, is where you'll want to begin.

Get a Little Closer

Whether it's a lighthearted sex game or the revelation of your deepest erotic dreams, sharing fantasies can bring you closer. You get to find out each other's sexiest secret wishes. Like eager teenagers on a first date, you find yourselves on a sexual adventure that takes you into territory far from your old sex routines. Your willingness to try new things (or at least talk about them) engenders trust. That's good for your relationship.

Our fantasies come from deep parts of ourselves When we share them, we're inviting another into our most private world. It's easy to feel emotionally exposed. You have to trust your partner to withhold judgment about your ability, performance, and (even scarier) your having these fantasies in the first place. Although these fears can be addressed largely by talking about them, moving past them takes willingness to extend trust and the cementing of that trust over time.

Not everyone is going to feel vulnerable sharing and trying out their fantasies. Some will be empowered; most will feel free at last to truly express themselves sexually; and many others will enjoy the verbal fantasy fuck of discussing their nastiest dreams out loud. Letting your fantasies run wild not only makes for pivotal sexual experiences, it can make your sexual relationship strong, vibrant, and alive.

Many people find emotional intimacy incredibly sexy. Couples in long-term relationships often discover that adding fantasies and role play to their sexual routine opens up a whole new universe of satisfying sex, forges a deep connection, and restores the energy of their relationship to the good ol' days of dating and courtship. If you and your partner play with fantasies as you would with a new sex toy, you can ignite some pretty potent erotic sparks.

Getting to Know Your Lover's Fantasies

Finding out what gets your lover's motor running is as simple—and possibly as nerve-wracking—as just asking. If you regularly talk about sex, this is much easier, but if sex isn't a typical topic for you, then you'll want to read this entire chapter before you go digging for erotic gold. If you're both fairly comfy with sex chat, ask your partner what some of their fantasies are, tell them some of yours, and watch the sparks begin to fly. Or you can each make a list of five sexual fantasies that interest you, and swap them. If your sweetie is a bit shy, but you can tell they're ripe for some new sex play, try looking for cues to what piques their interest—a scene in a film that had them holding their breath, a well-thumbed erotic novel on the nightstand—then ask them, in a sexy way, what they like about it.

Once you've got a fantasy theme in mind, you can begin to plan your scene. First, determine what the fantasy is, and who it belongs to. Is it your fantasy, is it your lover's, or both? If it's yours, you likely have all the fantasy components in your head, and all you need to do is tell your partner the details. If your ideas are too sketchy to put into words, see the fantasy suggestions in the first chapter—in fact, I recommend you read them together. Pick out the main elements—a sex act, an outfit, a role such as dominant or submissive—and tell your partner what it is about the fantasy that turns you on. Once you know who wants to do what, decide just how real you'd like that scenario to be. You can keep it in the realm of imagination, watching scenes in adult movies or reading erotic stories to each other that depict the fantasies that appeal to you. This way, your fantasy is a vicarious thrill, which is both incredibly hot on its own merits and great for nervous lovers. Also, you get the delight that comes from sharing your fantasy with your sweetie—or the heat of watching their face as they watch (or read) your number one turn-on.

You can take your fantasies a step further and bring hot talk into sex, where one partner describes the action of the fantasy in detail for the other. It's as if you're providing background narration as you go about your usual sex routine. You don't have to sound like a diva or a moaning, groaning porn star to describe your fantasies during sex. Remember that your lusty listener is going to be concentrating on the content of your words, not the inflection or the quality of your voice. Allow yourself to really sink into the story, and feel free to fill up the airtime; this is one time being a motormouth is to your advantage.

Don't know what to say? Describe exactly what you're doing, or what your partner is doing, in as much detail as possible. Allow your descriptions of in-the-moment sex to flower into a scene you know they'll like. For instance, if you're sitting on his face and simultaneously stroking his cock, describe the scene as though there were two of you doing these things to him. Voilà—instant fantasy threesome! Learn all about dirty talk, how to do it, and ideas for what to say in Chapter 6, "Weaving a Spell."

Sexy Surprises

Slow seductions and jointly-planned fantasies are among life's exquisite pleasures, but surprising your sweetie with something you know they'd like makes for an unforgettable sexual tryst. Make sure your partner has *some* idea that something's coming. Check in to make sure they're not exhausted, having a bad day, or will wish they'd showered before seeing you. Plan ahead for a successful surprise. Shop, get keys, wear the right outfit (or nothing at all).

- Surprise your partner with a light erotic treat such as an "aphrodisiac" dinner or a full-body erotic massage, or read a sexy story (possibly one with your favorite fantasy elements included).
- Slip them a note saying what you want to do with them later. Then do it.
- Leave a sexy present hinting at what's to come— tuck your panties into their pocket, pass them a note with instructions, leave an erotic picture where they'll find it, or bookmark an erotic story you want them to read.

The Sex Buffet

Sexual decadence comes in many forms, but perhaps the headiest and most sensual dining experiences happen when you make your lover into a tasty treat. Drizzle chocolate sauce, honey, or raspberry syrup, or slather whipped cream onto any part of the body that begs to be licked. Nibble on pieces of fruit you've placed on their body, slip a tasty morsel over his genitals and then eat it in full view. Set a meal (especially finger food like sushi) on your partner's quivering, excited torso and take your sweet time eating your fill. Just be sure to avoid getting sugars in her vagina, and don't insert any food anally (ever). Read more about messy fun in Chapter 11, "Sex Games."

- Surprise them with aggressive sex, or by enacting one of their fantasy sex acts (such as anal sex).

- If you live together, greet your partner when they get home wearing a fantasy outfit you know they'll like, or have one prepared for them to change into. You can be in lingerie, a schoolgirl outfit, house-cleaning in the nude, "caught" getting out of the shower (or watching porn, reading a dirty book, doing what you're not supposed to).

- Change your appearance in a sexy way, by wearing erotic undergarments or shaving your genitals. Try going out on a date wearing no underwear, and tell your partner during dinner.

- Use any of the techniques in later chapters to give your lover a surprise such as a striptease or lap dance (Chapter 6), a sudden spanking or punishment (Chapter 10), or improvised erotic role play (Chapter 4).

Talking to Your Partner

Erotic ideas can blossom into a shared fantasy as easily as making a wish—as long as you make that wish out loud. You and your partner may "click" sexually, sharing many of the same fantasies. Still, you have to say what you want. You might receive a mixed reply—part curiosity, part apprehension. A few folks will be met with a reluctance to even talk about fantasies, and some might meet an outright refusal.

Either way, for you to explore an idea together, one of you has to be bring it up—easy if you talk about sex regularly in your relationship, daunting if you never do. Whatever your situation, telling your partner you want to try something new can feel stressful—and if your fantasy makes *you* uncomfortable, this is an understatement. In fact, even thinking about talking about sex is stressful, sometimes!

If you have what you consider a tried-and-true style of sex, telling your partner that you want something to change is scary, and starting a conversation about your desire to experiment sexually can make you feel vulnerable. This is especially true with sexual fantasies that you enjoyed before you met your present partner. Opening yourself up and asking for something you want takes courage—but it also gives you an opportunity to learn more about what your lover likes and dislikes. Plus you might actually get what you want!

Before you tell all, put yourself in your partner's shoes: If the two of you don't normally talk about sex, and then suddenly one of you wants to, it might be upsetting—at first. Your lover may wonder if you've had sexual secrets all along. It's also very likely that your opening up this erotic treasure trove will give your partner the opportunity to tell you what's on their mind about sex, too.

Think about how you might bring up the subject in a way that would feel safe for you: Would you feel comfortable watching a movie with a scene that resembles your fantasy, and commenting on it after the show? Or do you think you'd feel more secure waiting until you are entwined in an intimate cuddle and then asking your partner what they think about trading fantasies? Another technique you can try is stating that you want to confess a fantasy—a sexual one—and that he or she doesn't have to reply right away. Tell them that you can have a conversation about it later; this gives both of you time to let the idea settle.

Consider ways in which you can encourage your partner to hear you out. Ask them to suspend judgment until you can explain how much fun you think the two of you will have—and how important their participation is to you. Be sure to reassure him or her that you find them incredibly sexy, and that the conversation wouldn't be happening unless you felt safe enough to reveal your deepest desires. Your lover needs to hear that they are the star of your show—and that you're ready to become closer than you've ever been before. The most important thing to think through beforehand is how you are going to make your partner feel safe. Mentally rehearse what you'd like to say before you actually have the conversation. Think about how your partner might react, so that you will be prepared to follow whichever route the discussion might take.

When Your Lover Is Reluctant

For a variety of reasons, your lover may not want to try out your sexual fantasy. Or your partner may want to make you happy but simply not understand what to do or what your fantasy means to you. Understanding these concerns can be helpful in having a constructive conversation about your partner's hesitations, learning how to overcome fears that might hold one of you back, and resolving what to do when one person feels okay about a fantasy while the other doesn't.

If your lover wants to try something sexually that you're afraid of, unsure about, or have a moral concern with, it can bring up powerful feelings. Adding any new sexual behavior to a relationship can feel like a make-or-break situation, and sometimes it is. Asking to try styles of expressing sexual intimacy can push your relationship to higher levels, or it can bring up so many issues that it rocks the boat—sometimes a little too hard. When fantasies make someone feel insecure, unsure of a partner's motivations, or profoundly uncomfortable, these issues can hit you at the core. This is especially true with fantasies related to degradation, fear, gender, age, or abuse.

When your own sexual fantasy makes you uncomfortable or offends you (and, confusingly, arouses you at the same time), you might worry that somewhere inside lurks a bad person, a person who "deserves" something harmful—or worse, that you actually want your fantasy to come true. Rape and incest fantasies are not uncommon, yet are extremely disturbing to contemplate. These fantasies are just that—fantasies—and so they will remain, in the realm of imagination or in the safety of fantasy play with someone you absolutely trust. Simply having a fantasy doesn't mean you want to see it enacted in reality.

Ready to Play?

Now you're ready to play! Fantasies about simple sex acts, with basic scenarios, can be played out whenever you're both ready, and wherever you like. Just be sure that you have privacy. Home is the best place to act out your fantasies, and with a little hot talk and imagination, imaginary sex partners can join in, you can shift the time and place however you want, and you're free to use sex toys, fetish objects, and props to add to your arousal.

Set aside time when you'll both be free of distractions and can really relax—turn off your phones, make sure your roommates are really away, send the kids to a sitter. Make sure you've shopped for props and accessories, such as a dog collar, whipped cream, massage oil, full-length mirror. (Don't forget your naughty imagination!) Have these items ready ahead of time, or if you're visiting your lover's house, bring your treats with you. Most importantly, bring a sense of sexual adventure and a sense of humor, because fantasy play is exactly that—play.

Not Tonight

BY ALISON TYLER

Sounds silly, I guess, but sometimes when I see him, I don't want to fuck him, I want to *be* him. Matt has the perfect male body, in my opinion. Broad shoulders, a long, lean torso, slim hips, and an awesome ass. He has a deeply fuckable body, and I do love to fuck him. But sometimes I don't want him to climb on top of me and pound into me, don't want him to bend me over and take me from behind, don't want him to press me up against the wall and make me writhe with pleasure.

No, what I want is to slide inside him and see the world from within his head. And I want to devour some summertime chicklet dolled up in one of those swishy floral dresses and tie-up espadrilles and fuck *her* while being him.

Too much like that John Malkovich movie?

Maybe.

But why can't I be him? Just for an evening. Or even for an hour. Why can't *I* be the one to move through the crowd and pick up a girl, any girl? (He can have any girl.) Why can't I take one home, or out to some back alley, and push her up against the brick wall out there, tear her panties down and fuck her?

That's all I want. One hour. One hour inside his body so that I can find out what it's like—not just to be a man, but to be *him*. I want to manhandle my throbbing cock, to hold it, to fondle it. I want to force-feed every inch of it to some pretty girl, to make her drink me, and drain me. To make her feel my power.

He's not always that type, I know. He is sweet and caring and gentle. He is monogamous and dedicated to me. But I'd be that type if I were him. I'd be the type to control the situation. I'd be the type to take charge. It would feel good to take charge. God, it would feel amazing.

I get to a point where I am all-consumed by the thought. So I take one step forward, or really one roll forward on the mattress, and I curl my body up next to his in bed, and I say, "I have a fantasy…"

He slides one strong arm around me, holding me close. "Tell me, baby," he whispers back, the way he always does. He likes my mind best. More than my ripe, lush breasts. More than my thick, black hair. More than the curves of my hips or the swell of my ass, he likes my thoughts. My dirty fantasies. My X-rated visions. "Tell me where your mind is going tonight," he croons in his low, husky voice.

"I want…" I start, but I can't say it.

"Tell me."

"No," I whisper, shaking my head.

"Tell," he says, and his voice is insistent.

"I'll show you," I decide. Because that will work best.

"Show—" he starts, but I put my finger to his lips, and without another word, I climb out of bed and grab the satchel containing my outfit and all my recently purchased gear, and I disappear into our bathroom. I can almost hear his thoughts going crazy in the other room—*Where is she going? What's she doing?*—but I pay more attention to my own thoughts. At this point, they're all that matter.

I gaze at myself as I bind my breasts flat with an Ace bandage. I admire my body as I slip into my new harness and adjust my fine, handsome cock. I slide into the faded 501s, put on the boots, and add a wife-beater T-shirt that makes my arms look cut and fierce.

Who am I?

Will he know?

I gel my hair and tuck my ponytail up into a cap, then slip on a pair of his shades. I can see it. I can feel it. I add cologne, from the expensive bottle I bought him last Christmas, and then I walk back into our bedroom and wait to see what his response will be.

"Oh, Jesus," he says when he sees me, and I know with that ripple of pleasure that runs instantly through me that he's game. "Oh, *god*," he says, looking me up and down. I'm tall and lean and hard. My hand is already on my belt. I want to undress as quickly as I wanted to dress. But first, I have to strip him down. I have to oil him up. I have to kiss him all over, lovely flower that he is. Because now that I'm him, well, who does *he* have to be?

We don't need to answer that question, do we? I didn't think so.

Even though I feel like being naked so he can really see the transformation, I don't take off my clothes this time. I need him too fast for that. I part my jeans and let him admire my cock. I manhandle my cock, my fist wrapped tight. I want to slide it across his pretty lips. I want to watch him deep-throat it.

He wants that, too.

"Look," I say. "Get close so you can see me. Really see me."

He scrambles on the bed to obey. His mouth is open before I can command it. I don't have to tell him what to do. His lips part, and he takes me in. I feel him pulling on my cock. I feel how hungry he is for that. I envision him draining me, taking me all the way to climax with the sucking motions of his ravenous mouth.

Later. *After.*

For now, I push him back. There's lube in the drawer by the bed. Usually, it's lube for me. Now, it's lube for him. I tell him to get me the bottle, and then I let him watch me grease myself up.

"You know where this is going," I say, seeing his eyes widen, seeing him bite hard on his bottom lip, as if he might want to say something, but doesn't quite dare. "You know where," I say, softer, but I can tell from the rosy blush on his face that he understands. Of course he does. Then I roughly roll him over, pull his boxers off, spread those lovely asscheeks of his, and kiss him there. Mmm. I take my time, the way he takes his time, and I can tell he is growing more aroused from the way he shifts against the sheets.

He likes this. My baby likes this.

I oil him up, so gently, so sweetly, my fingers going deep inside him, and while I work them slowly into his asshole, I press my face against his smooth skin and breathe in deep. Oh, is he sweet. He is my angel. My lover. My sweet young thing in a floral dress and tie-up espadrilles, so ready and willing to get fucked against some back-alley wall.

I sit up on my haunches, and I get ready to plunge. My baseball cap comes off, but my hair stays in place, and I'm still him as I work the first part of my thick, ready cock into his asshole.

And as I fuck him, I realize that we've blurred, because there I am in the mirror. There I am. But who am I? And there he is, his expression one of awe and surrender. And who is he? And more important than either of those questions is this one: Does it matter?

No. Not at all.

Not tonight.

Role Play

It could be that your Halloween outfit inspires you long past October. Or your partner might confess attraction to a TV or movie character or celebrity. You may have any number of fantasy sources from memories, porn movies, books—you name it. Perhaps in your fantasies you're a naughty schoolgirl about to be punished by a handsome male teacher. Or maybe you're a patient at the hospital administered to by a sexy nurse who deems your best treatment to be oral stimulation. Perhaps you have a repeat fantasy that you've shared with your lover—you visit a darkened movie theater and perform oral sex on the first stranger you encounter—and your lover wants to make it come true, but without any risk. In your erotic daydreams, are you a lost tourist who wanders into a secret sex club—and is made a slave?

Have you and your lover shared a role-playing fantasy that you'd like to try? Can you really make all these fantasies come true, safely and sanely? When you learn the basics of role play, yes, you certainly can!

Erotic Adult Theater for Two

Erotic role play, where two or more people adopt roles to act out a fantasy, is a terrific way to add spice and exciting variation to your usual sexual routines. Role play, because you tap into your shared fantasies, takes an already great sex life and makes it extraordinary, gives it new dimension, and adds playfulness—or intensity—to your intimacy. Trying out fantasy scenarios, much like playing an explicit adult version of "make believe," can be like a sex toy you bring into the bedroom (or harem, doctor's office, schoolroom...). And as with other sex toys, some couples will use role-play now and then to mix things up, while others will enjoy it as a regular part of their rich sexual panorama.

Some fantasies you may wish to explore will star doctors, firemen, nurses, or anyone in a sexy uniform. Many fantasies will revolve around subtle—or overt—dominance and submission themes, as for example when someone finds donning a stern demeanor arousing or has erotic daydreams about surrendering to authority figures. You may find yourself drawn to act out fully-formed scenes that are as far away from reality as possible, taking place on other planets, in other times, or in settings that would be illogical—or dangerous—in real life. Let the erotic fantasies you already enjoy shape your role-playing scenarios. There is no one right way to role-play. Because role play is fueled by your imagination, you don't need to buy a new wardrobe, hunt down perfect props, create fake accents, stay in character every minute, carry off the whole thing by yourself, or learn terminology or rules. Unless you want to, that is: Some people find that wearing the perfect outfit makes it all that much hotter, that props heighten the erotic tension, or that an accent makes it more fun. Because, after all, role play is just the same as playing make believe as a child—it's play between two people who want to enjoy the possibilities within a given scenario. And while toy guns made playing cowgirl more vivid, being held at "fingerpoint" always worked just as well.

In erotic role play, you and your partner(s) choose a scenario with erotic potential, and go from there. One of you will gravitate to a particular role—the choice usually comes from a strong attraction to a particular icon or type of behavior. How far you go with setting, costumes, props, and character is up to you.

Waiting in the Wings

Start out with dirty talk, explicit banter leading up to sex or during sex. You can describe a fantasy (even closing your eyes if you feel more comfortable), confess a scenario that turns you on, or simply describe or exaggerate what you're both currently doing. Mine your partner's responses for clues about what will work in role play. If he gets excited when you call him a "bad boy," push the envelope and ask him *how* he's been bad. Develop his perspective by egging him on and expand your persona in ways that fit his erotic world.

Nervous about taking the scene from the imagination to the verbal? Start by practicing alone. Talk dirty to a mirror. Don't worry about feeling silly; remember that your companion will be a willing partner in escaping to your shared fantasy—and when you do it, it will be in context.

When you get your banter going, focus on describing details, such as the way the dog collar looks, feels, and how the buckles sparkle in the light. If you are still shy about talking explicitly in a face-to-face encounter, begin with an email exchange or a telephone conversation. Easing into role-playing with dirty talk can be even easier when you read your partner an erotic short story—and suggest enacting the best parts.

If you find it hard to come up with things to say, remember that role-playing is much like erotic theater: Your role will give you the framework for your motivation and language. Props and other elements of theater may actually make it easier. For example, a highway patrol officer "arresting" a reckless driver may feel more convincing once the cuffs are on.

When you venture beyond dirty talk and add developed roles, outfits, props, and scenarios, it's very important to make sure that each of you is clear about the other's expectations. She might want to be a naughty schoolgirl, hoping to be reprimanded for being sexually promiscuous with a perverted teacher, while you may think she's naughty because she's seducing a hapless teacher—two very different scenarios and with very different power dynamics. Talking about the scenario beforehand won't ruin it or give away the good parts, because you can't predict how the scenario will play out or how turned on you might get. But make sure you get the outcome you crave (and find yourself in the predicament you desire) by giving your role-play partner specifics about what turns you on within the context of the scene. You may find it helpful to write down your ideas before you have your conversation.

Erotic Acting

Now it's time for the librarian to let down her hair—or pin it up tight and put on those sexy glasses. Being a good erotic actor might seem daunting at first, but all it takes is enthusiasm and erotic desire. If you really want to be doing it, you'll push past any "stage fright" and let lust and passion for your lover lead you through your role-play scenes. While it might seem odd to consider, out of the blue, donning a pirate costume, affecting a swagger, and trying to keep a straight face while man-handling your wench's "booty," when the action starts, you may find you feel less awkward than you would think. Any role you play will have an element of your-self in it, somewhere, that you can draw from. Of course, if a role sounds like a ridiculous idea, or you just don't think you can pull it off, you don't have to do it—or you can negotiate with your lover a variation that's comfortable for you and meets everyone's needs.

If you're drawn to role play with someone you're attracted to, and the scenario turns you on, getting into the part is the step that may seem the most daunting. Costumes, accessories, and setting up a room to reflect the scene will help immeasurably by placing you in the right atmosphere—sometimes this is done simply with a single item such as a stethoscope, whip, knife, hand-cuffs, panties, collar, or dog bowl.

Think about your role for a minute—playing that role for your lover turns you on, so evidently something in it resonates with you. What is it? How does your role express itself—stern, cold, nervous (that one's easy!), excited, horny, petulant, selfish, frightened, angry, demure? A sizzling sexpot beneath your cool exterior, or a nervous virgin who wants only to please? Give yourself room to have several feelings at once, mingling your real-life emotions with those of your character. Roles tend to fall into two general categories: If you're in the more active role, you'll want to get something sexual from your lover, while in the receptive role you'll be reacting to your partner's innuendo, sexual dominance, or advances. Whatever role you take, let your own erotic desire be your primary motivating factor.

Motivation is why you're there—as yourself and as the character you're playing. Your goal is always to turn on your lover and yourself, and for both of you to have a great time getting off in a new, exciting, and sexually significant way. But the role or character you are personifying also has his or her own motivation. Your character's goal may be to humiliate, punish, or control your partner's character. Your interaction with your partner will be primarily sexual, but different from the role or persona you're used to playing with this person (though not *too* different than you'd like it to be).

Say, for instance, you've been asked to play a sexy teacher who spanks the mischievous schoolboy, and you don't normally spank your boyfriend in your sexual routines. You'll probably find that once you put on your teacher's outfit part of you gets an erotic charge out of erotically dominating your boyfriend—or you wouldn't have agreed to try the scenario. If you're still feeling uncertain but are willing to play along with the sexual fun and games, you can tap into your eagerness to serve up your lover's number one sexual fantasy on a silver platter—and give him what he deserves, because you know how much it means to him, and how much it turns him on.

There's nothing wrong with allowing yourself to really get into "punishing" your partner, especially if you find it makes your shared sex life exciting. Don't worry about feeling silly—if you do, laugh it up and then get down to business. You can have fun, feel goofy, and get off all at once. If you're worried about your performance, or anything else, remember that the role-play scenario is just a momentary, fun thing that you're trying: A little experimentation is just that; it's not a commitment. Before you begin, do whatever you need to get into role—read erotica, watch porn, play music, dress in costume. It's extremely helpful to be aroused when you "make your entrance" into the scene. Masturbating a little or touching yourself erotically before the scene begins will turn you on and help take the edge off any fear you might be holding on to—plus it gives you the proper motivation!

Plan It, Janet

There is a whole world of sexual expression and adventure around the corner when you add planning, details, and surprises to your scenario. That stripper fantasy will be even hotter with the purchase of a red vinyl bustier, and your partner's eyes will pop out of their head when you set your room up as a stage for a lap dance. That Halloween police uniform will be much more effective if you have a pair of mirrored sunglasses, and the experience will be unforgettable if you "arrest" him on the hood of his car—even if it's parked safely in the garage.

Once you've made your fantasies and expectations clear to each other, and covered what both of you *don't* want to include, you'll have a better idea of what to wear, how to accessorize, and the ideal setting for your scene. With this information, you can plan the logistics of your scene.

Make a date and set a time with a realistic window, allowing for the fantasy to run for at least an hour. You'll want plenty of time for the fantasy to play itself out. Let it go on as long as possible—this makes for a more effective scene and a lasting impression. Make sure that no one will interrupt you—your roommates are definitely gone, the kids are away—and unplug the phone. You don't want any distractions or interruptions to jar you from your fantasy, or run the risk of having to explain your private lives to anyone. If your fantasy might include loud music, the unmistakable sounds of paddling or whipping, or escalate to yelling, be sure to have your windows and doors closed, be sure the neighbors are at work, or have a cover story ready in case someone checks in on you.

Stock your "play" area with plenty of water (stay hydrated!), any sex toys you might want, lube, towels, and props. Give yourself plenty of time to relax afterward, as well. Have some snacks and tasty beverages waiting for you—if your scene is successful, it'll feel good to recharge, and if things don't go as you planned or hoped, you'll have some nourishment to help you regroup.

Surprise scenes should be planned out carefully, and the person being surprised should always have some idea about what's coming—even if they don't know exactly when. What if you deck your apartment out as the set of *Star Trek*, don your Klingon makeup, and she comes home upset and exhausted from an awful day at work? Let your partner know you want to plan a fantasy surprise, and tell them which role-playing scenario you have in mind. Ask when your partner will be available to play, but tell them you ultimately want it to remain a surprise. Suggest a few dates, such as Wednesday, Thursday, or Friday evening. It's also okay to give your partner an assigned date and time to come over, or to meet you at a given location—in fact, you can erotically "command" them! Tell him or her to meet you at a certain café, in a secretary outfit, and surprise them with a job interview. Then adjourn to your "office." Turn an ordinary meeting into a special evening by asking them to come over and mentioning that you need a "repairman" to fix your sink—hint, hint.

Some surprise scenes will take careful negotiation, especially if they involve force or implied violence, being out in public, or other partners. Be sure to read more about negotiation in Chapter 3, public sex in Chapter 8, real and implied force in Chapter 10, and adding partners in Chapter 5.

Public role play—especially in everyday roles—can be a secret thrill that you both share, right in front of everyone. For instance, you can pretend to meet a total stranger (actually your lover), carry out a seduction, then adjourn for sex elsewhere, complete with witnesses to cement your roles. Or you can take the roles a bit further, impersonating a job applicant in an interview, a sex worker picking up a client, or someone really famous (a porn star!) picking up a groupie for a little casual sex.

Be sure you choose your roles wisely. Don't put yourself in a position where your boyfriend may be late and you actually are mistaken for a real sex worker, and the hotel staff calls the police because you are soliciting in their lobby. Don't be caught enacting any scenarios that may get you in trouble, such as pretend abductions or age play (where one of you plays an obviously underage character). And don't charge into the 7-Eleven in your sorcerer robes to use your mind control powers on the pretty wench in the candy aisle, even if she's your wife.

Classic Roles

It's one thing to have an idea already in your head, but sometimes it's nice to glean new ideas to stir the pot. Once you decide on an appealing role or scenario, where do you go from there? You can flesh out your characters with the descriptions of classic scenarios below—let the characters' motivations inspire you to action.

Boss

Corporate authority figures dress impeccably and have big desks, notepads, and briefcases, phones that need answering, dictation that needs taking, and they often have to work late hours. The pressure is immense, and they require reliable help. When interviewing prospective staff they usually need to find out what the applicant is capable of, and the promise of sexual favors in exchange for getting the job is a strong incentive. Bosses like to give dictation to their secretaries while letting their hands wander, punish bad receptionists for improper dress or attitude with clients, blackmail workers for sex, search employees for stolen Post-Its and pens, and check for appropriate undergarments.

Cat Burglar, Criminal, Biker

Outfits include tight, form-fitting, all-black cat suits with masks, gloves, and boots, "thug" attire, biker leathers (vests, chaps, sunglasses, bandanas, fake tattoos), and stockings over the face. Burglars, criminals, and thieves have sacks of loot and rope (for climbing or binding), can possess fighting abilities, may sneak up from behind or hide in the bedroom, ride into town on loud bikes and "take" what they want, or can be caught in the act of stealing or being bad. They may trade sex for freedom, may take sexual favors as easily as a precious jewel, put you over their bike and have their way with you, or just make great anonymous lovers in darkened rooms, alleys, or rooftops. Cops like to catch criminals, know what I mean?

Cheerleader, Football Captain

The uniform may come out of mothballs, from an authentic online resource, thrift store, Halloween store, or stripper outlet, but they remain the same: Cheerleaders have short skirts, pom-poms, pig- or ponytails, little white socks; football players have jerseys or letterman jackets. Cheerleaders can be sexually inexperienced or very experienced, looking for a ride home, dressing in the locker room, showering with other cheerleaders, under the bleachers, in the backseat of a car after the big game. Football players can be boys seeing how far they can get, nervous virgins, frisky in the locker room, caught masturbating under the bleachers, or attacked by a vicious group of cheerleaders.

Doctor, Nurse

Classic doctors and nurses wear white uniforms, unless they're in surgeon's scrubs. They might have stethoscopes, gloves, tongue depressors, glasses, a clipboard, or various sexual examination tools including speculum and lubricant. A butt plug can easily pass as your rectal thermometer. Doctors and nurses examine patients, take notes, ask questions both proper and inappropriate, test sexual response, give sponge baths, and take samples of tissue and body fluids.

Hero, Heroine, Firefighter

Professional heroes such as firefighters wear uniforms, while others may be ordinary citizens who romantically save you when you're in danger. They are fearless and strong, and in these scenes, large objects can be lifted and victims carried to safety, where they are lovingly cared for with massage, medical treatment, bathing, and sensuous sex. Conversely, heroes may find the sexual attraction so intense that before you are even rescued you rip each other's clothes off, danger be damned.

Human Dog, Pony, Pet

If your fantasy is being a good kitty, bad doggie, pony in need of training, or any other type of animal, you can dress in your regular clothing, a costume, or nothing at all. Many animals require collars and some require leashes, while others like ponies may need bridles, saddles (or simply blankets, as pony gear is expensive), horsehair butt plugs, and a riding crop. Animals can be trained, reprimanded, punished for not going on the paper, made to drink from bowls on the floor, petted and played with, groomed and washed and fed treats. They can behave well or be naughty, scratching and biting, being affectionate and licking, rolling around, humping furniture and legs—or people!

Military Uniforms

These command respect—and they look incredibly sexy. Generals, majors, sergeants, and privates, Army, Navy, Air Force, Special Forces, Marines—call in the troops and let the good times roll. Outfits for military fantasies are easy to put together, and a trip to a military surplus store can have you set for turning your bedroom into boot camp by nightfall. With military scenarios you train new recruits, give or take orders, break the rules after "lights out," go on dangerous missions, save each other from danger, seduce civilians, take prisoners, or any other salacious fantasy that real servicepersons would get in a lot of trouble for.

Multiple Partners

When you want to play around with the possibility of threesomes, foursomes, or orgies, you and your partner can role-play as if others are in the room by running porn in the background, incorporating sex toys as extra penises and vaginas, and even switching roles completely. A "pretend" gang bang is enhanced when the receptive party is blindfolded; blindfolds make an effective cover for a partner as shoving dildos into their mouth as they penetrate them simultaneously elsewhere. This technique also works well in "sexual slavery" scenarios—for example, where one party "makes" the other give fellatio to imaginary participants.

Pimp

Pimps and hustlers can be of either gender, and their sexual chattel can be women, men, trannies—anyone

Where to Shop?

Just where do you get your gear? The Resources chapter at the end of this book is organized by topic, making specifics easy to find. For special outfits, many people scope out their local costume shops or save up money and wait for Halloween to roll around, stocking up on costumes and accessories to last them year-round. Uniform, medical, and army supply stores will sell to the public if you want realism, and stores catering to strippers and drag queens can be found in most major cities. Get creative—make costumes and accessories, get ideas for setting the scene from movies and books, and don't be afraid to go to the fabric store to purchase fake fur to drape on your bed for your *Clan of the Cave Bear* scene!

the pimp fancies. Pimps have money and style, though it's an exaggerated style that often becomes a campy costuming experience—big hats, gold chains, big rings, flashy suits: Use your imagination. Pimps persuade their moneymaking staff with sex, coercion, and, of course, by "breaking them in." They can be rough or gentle, smooth or streetwise. This role works especially well with an opposite, such as the "innocent" street urchin, or for twice the fun, the police officer.

Police

Officers are clad in dark-blue uniforms with shiny badges, leather belts, and polished shoes. They can have mirrored shades, utility belts, handcuffs, nightsticks, clipboards, and hats. (Fake guns are for indoor, private play only; in public, a fake gun can produce a tragic response from onlookers). Cops can stop suspects, ask tough questions, become suspicious about alibis, frisk and search, cuff and rough up, intimidate, threaten, and exact sexual favors.

Priest, Nun

Outfits for these icons are most easily obtained at Halloween, and once suited up, it's time for confession! These roles can be either proper (and then seduced) or debauched (and decadent). The priest or nun might hear confessions, force a few Hail Marys out of you, administer spankings, help you find the proper position for worship, lose their virginity, flagellate themselves or others for impure thoughts, or seek other priests/nuns for sexual solace.

Prostitute, Sex Worker

Prostitutes, high-class call girls, escorts, strippers, and erotic masseuses can dress in a variety of sexy outfits, from trashy to classy, and especially clothing that is revealing. Streetwalkers will go for wigs, short skirts, no underwear, heavy makeup, high heels, and a small purse with condoms in it. Strippers and masseuses can wear less, opting for lingerie, wigs, and heels—g-strings and straps make a good place to put tips. Expensive "dates" wear suitably expensive evening or business wear. All sex workers will want to have lube on hand. Your motivation will be to please your client, and you can name your menu of activities and charges, and your limits—then go beyond them for that "special" customer.

Repairman, Deliveryman

Showing up at someone's door to deliver a special package or to fix a broken drain requires an outfit that represents your job and profession. Delivery personnel will want brown shirts and shorts, or navy blue shorts and a crisp white shirt—plus a cap, a clipboard, and a parcel. Repair people will need work clothes, a badge or patch bearing someone's name, and plenty of tools—wrenches, lube, sex toys. They can invite themselves in, be seduced by horny housewives (or househusbands), make advances, demand sexual favors as payment, or be caught masturbating in the bathroom.

Rock Star, Actor

What do you wear when you're a rock star? Whatever you want, but usually something casually glamorous, like leather pants and a T-shirt, though it's good to take your inspiration from a rock star your lover finds sexy. Same with famous actors—wear a typical outfit of whichever TV or film actor your sweetie finds the sexiest, because the key in making these fantasies hot is to provide special access to the working star. A backstage pass, visit to a trailer, groupie sex, dressing-room debauchery—it's all what's for dinner. Famous people can be sexual users, aggressive seducers, be swept off their feet by gorgeous fans, stay in stage character, or play around with their TV or big-screen producers.

School Authority Figures

These people dress properly in adult attire, such as a suit and tie, governess costume, nun's habit, janitor uniform, or gym-teacher attire with shorts and a whistle. They can have chalk, blackboards, pens, clipboards, assignments, a janitor's closet and brooms, locker room showers to frolic in, paddles, rulers, or dunce caps. School authority figures can punish, be seduced by students, take advantage of situations, extract favors for grades, give impossible assignments, give rides home from school, or grill students about their sexual experiences.

Schoolgirl, Boy

Adult schoolkids will wear uniforms such as plaid Catholic-school skirts and white shirts with ties, or other youthful outfits, depending on the age they're portraying. Accessories might include apples, pens and pencils, binders, glasses—or things they're not supposed to have like cigarettes, condoms, porn, lipstick, alcohol, or missing underwear. They can be good and innocent, or naughty and experienced, or anything in between. They might be tardy, in trouble for cutting class, caught cheating—and they usually get spanked, and more. They might play opposite teachers and principals, nuns, older people outside school, babysitters, stepparents, older boy- or girlfriends.

Secretary

Office personnel—or applicants for office jobs—will want to dress their professional best (unless they want to be punished). Slacks, a skirt, dressy shoes (nothing too slutty unless you want trouble) white shirt, tie, glasses, hair in neat presentation, clean-shaven, light makeup, and no underwear are all recommended. A steno pad and pencil are good props, as are résumés, briefcases, and freshly typed letters full of typos in need of a boss's (dis)approval. Secretaries may be desperate for a job, can be the office slut, the "new girl," trying to please the boss, just doing her job, or simply enjoying the view from beneath the desk. You will often be required to work after hours.

Sleazy Photographer or Pornographer

Like the pimp, these characters dress sleazily, with chains, open shirts, polyester slacks, white shoes, and comb-overs. They like to wear sunglasses indoors, and their motivation is to convince their subjects to take off their clothes and perform sexually for the camera. Good props are cameras, both still and digital, and if your bud-get allows, Polaroids and video cameras so both of you will have keepsakes from the experience. Great for cou-ples who want to experiment with erotic photography or making their own dirty movies, because often it's eas-ier *not* to be yourself for the first few times in front of the cameras.

Stranger

Role-playing a stranger is one of the easiest, most excit-ing ways to play with a lover. The stranger can dress any way he or she likes, in usual attire or something totally out of the ordinary. You can meet anywhere—bars, restaurants, movie theaters, on the bus or train, shopping, in a make-believe setting at home, or anywhere else that sounds fun. Set a loose time to "meet" your stranger and publicly flirt, tease, and seduce each other. Don't you wonder what passersby will think? All you need to do is act as if you've never touched or known this person intimately in your life, and the resulting sex will be unlike any you've ever had. Make sure you meet somewhere that is convenient to a private locale for sex, such as near your home or at a hotel bar (especially suitable for playing out-of-town businessperson and sex worker).

Victim, Patient

Being saved from danger by a sexy hero, firefighter, police officer, requires no special outfit, unless you want to play up your situation with torn clothing and fake injuries. Patients may dress as usual, with no apparent injuries, or may opt for bandages that need changing, fake cuts and bruises, and makeshift dressings. Patients in hospital scenarios will want to wear a hospital gown—a garment likely invented by someone with a dirty mind. Of course, your ailment is probably sexual, and you may require relief treatment, or treatment suited to relieve your attendant. Then again, medical care is expensive and you may want to settle your bill on the spot.

Gender Play

Have you ever wondered what it would be like having sex as the opposite gender? Probably everyone has, at one time or another, and for some people trying out this idea with a lover may be their number one, red-hot fantasy. Playing around with gender might be something you've contemplated once or twice, or fancy as a new idea, or it might be a fantasy so intense that you consider it a sort of sexual and emotional "home"—familiar, reliable, and sublime. Gender play can be as simple as a man wearing lipstick, or as ritualized as a woman undergoing a complete make-over to effectively pass as a man.

For some, the area of gender play can be somewhat frightening and uncomfortably challenging to their ideas about their own identities. Others don't see it that way at all, but simply as another playful sex game to share with an adventurous lover. Still others embrace the challenge to their sexual identity, allowing the gender transformation to create new configurations that are much more comfortable for them than their original manifestations.

Wearing the clothing and adopting the mannerisms of the opposite sex will not turn you into the opposite sex, make you gay or lesbian, change who you are attracted to, or alter how you identify sexually. Nor will it show you what it's really like to be the opposite sex. It does not mean you are transsexual or transgender, though for those individuals it might be a step toward feeling comfortable with who they really are.

If your lover wants to cross-dress for sex, suspend your judgment and ask what the turn-on is—and how you can heighten the experience. You might find that "playing lesbian" with your boyfriend (who dresses for the occasion in your best Bebe gear) is a total turn-on. Or your partner might like to dress *you* up and pretend you are two gay men. If the idea of gender play upsets you, say so as openly as you can and explain why, if possible. It may be that you've always wanted to see your girlfriend dress like a man and treat you accordingly.

This may be confusing to her—she might wonder if you simply want to sleep with a man, which may not be not the case. (Even if you are interested in men sexually, in this scenario, you want to play with gender with your female partner.) Light gender play isn't a wish to become something you're not—it's a wish to have the best of both worlds in your bed.

Dressing for gender play runs along the spectrum of what is most erotic for you—some might want to "go all the way" while others prefer to play around with in-between measures, like boys in skirts and eyeliner, but no other feminine signifiers. Gender play for women might include a business suit, a biker outfit, jeans and wife-beater T-shirt, or any attire considered masculine and sexy. She could go with light makeup or none (simple lipstick is common), slicked-back hair, suspenders, men's underwear, dress shoes, or boots. She can wear false facial hair, no bra (or her breasts bound with an Ace bandage), and a strap-on. Get a good-quality harness and a dildo that is either suitable for "packing" (a softie) or a firmer model to be used for penetration or fellatio. Is your strap-on for sexual function, or gender play, or both?

Men can don women's undergarments, foundation wear such as corsets, stockings, lingerie. High heels in larger sizes, skirts, dresses, gowns, wigs, makeup, false eyelashes, anything that sounds erotically appealing will complete the experience. Perfume, lotions, nail polish, even shaving underarms and legs are all on the list of options, as is the technique of "tucking" the penis and testicles flat to the body to minimize the bulge (though for some the bulge under their skirt is a huge turn-on). Bras can be stuffed with whatever's handy, or you can purchase breast prostheses.

You can create any type of role-playing scene you like, combining characters and gender in any way that turns you on. Gender play can be a sexual "punishment," where one partner is mock-forced into drag. Or one partner can be caught trying on lipstick, boxer shorts, or anything else that's "illicit" and sounds like fun—be playful and imaginative in your scenarios.

Age Play

Role-playing significant age differences is a surprisingly common fantasy—everyone knows what an adult school-girl wears—though it's a fantasy with roots that may be disturbing for people who confuse fantasy with reality. Role-playing where one partner is much younger than the other does not mean that either party truly eroticizes young people. Those who molest children *do*. There is none of that dynamic in men who ask their girlfriends to play the older, sexually experienced babysitter, or in adult women who dress in school uniforms to play-act with their husbands.

Sometimes these fantasies can, however, bring up powerful issues for the consenting adults who enjoy them. For instance, while playing "daddy's little girl" with her lesbian lover, a woman might feel uncomfortable afterward with the associations, memories of past abuse, or personal meanings the fantasy brings up. Sexual fantasies are powerful because they have their roots in our subconscious and the oft-mysterious working of our libido. If you find that your age play or gender play scenarios wake up memories or feelings that disturb you, read about taking steps toward sexual healing in Staci Haines's *The Survivor's Guide to Sex*, or watch her video *Healing Sex: The Complete Guide to Sexual Wholeness*.

Many people are just fine with the incendiary results they get from age play scenarios—playing an inexperienced youth opposite an experienced older figure can be a turn-on like no other. Young roles allow us to be coy, innocent, bratty, curious, naughty, in need of discipline, protection, or tenderness. Boys and girls get spanked, groomed, dressed up (or undressed), taught the facts of life, seduced by older figures such as teachers, babysitters, strangers, friend's moms or dads—or, even more taboo, family members, authority figures, or clergy. They get to be "taken care of," and the feeling of not having to be in control is a blissful and incredibly arousing relief for many.

Playing older roles to your "younger" lover is a delightfully dirty way to lavish attention on your sweetie, and it appeals to the authority figure in all of us. Playing the seducer (or occasionally the one seduced or overtaken), the role allows you to be the "experienced" one, giving erotic instruction, calling the shots, and enjoying the make-believe of exploring an unfamiliar body. The scene may be intense, heated, and unbelievably arousing, or it can verge on hilarity as your husband claims to have "never done *that* before!"

5

Threesomes, Foursomes, and Moresomes

Is a threesome your number one fantasy? You're not alone— in fact, you're in the majority. When top-ten-fantasy lists are compiled, sex with multiple partners always tops the charts. Online surveys like www.askmen.com, glossy magazines such as *Men's Health* and *Cosmopolitan*, and popular women's true fantasy compilations, such as Nancy Friday's collections, all consistently list sex with more than one person as a widely popular fantasy.

Sex with multiple partners, in an array of alluring combinations, can be a mind-blowing experience for everyone involved. But despite its extraordinarily popularity as a fantasy, few people know how to make it happen in real life. Most threesomes and other unconventional groupings tend to be unplanned. A multiple-partner fantasy that "just happens" can be incredible—or it can be disappointing, or worse. It can bring you and your partner closer—or just rock the boat. Making a threesome happen, and having hot sex during the experience, all in a spirit of safety and fun, takes a bit more than chance and luck. For some couples, this is the ultimate sexual adventure, one where a bit of planning leaves everyone spent, satisfied, or hungry for more.

Three, Four, and More

Multiple-partner sex, where everyone is licking, sucking, fucking, and coming until all are satisfied, can truly be one of life's peak sexual experiences. Movies that depict a threesome as taboo make it all the more alluring, and nowhere is the threesome more common than in mainstream porn. Maybe you want to try a three-way to spice things up or to imitate a scene that turned you on in a video. You may want to satisfy a craving for same-sex contact (or opposite-sex pairings, in the case of lesbian and gay couples)—or you may just want to watch.

But how do you engineer more than two bodies coming together? Most often, a couple invites someone outside the relationship to participate in a sexual encounter: two women and one man, two men and one woman, three women, or three men. Allowing for transgender partners, the possible combinations multiply. Of course, three friends (or even strangers) can simply come together to have sex.

The arrangement of the encounter depends on the couple's fantasy, their rules and limits, and the third party's expectations. For instance, a female partner may want to have sex with her boyfriend and another woman primarily to focus on the other woman—while he assists but does not directly participate. This fulfills the girlfriend's fantasy of sex with another woman, the boyfriend's fantasy of being close while two women have sex, their shared fantasy of sex with a new partner, and the new partner's fantasy of sex with a woman while her boyfriend watches. Whew!

Your preferred arrangement may include a third person sharing the affection and sex within your established partnership as an equal participant. You and your partner may like to "take turns" with the newcomer. You might want to try something else, such as two men having sex with a woman and her strap-on, two women "using" a man as a sex toy, a couple having sex with an anonymous stranger, a woman watching her boyfriend and another man (or another woman), or any number of novel scenarios.

Foursomes are just what they sound like—a couple plus two more, often another couple. You can have opposite-sex couples, same-sex couples, or a mix of the two. Or a couple can invite two unrelated participants—though it helps if these newcomers have a desire to have sex with each other, as well. We usually think of a foursome as four people having sex together, but again, depending on limits and expectations, one or more may watch or assist rather than participate. Some people consider two couples simply having sex in the same room to be a foursome. (Remember prom night?) They can enjoy the added excitement of watching each other; even without sexual contact, it's a hot slice of voyeurism.

Add a person and you've got a threesome, couple up and you've got a foursome, add more than two to your twosome, and you've got…quite a party. Sex with many partners is another big fantasy that couples share. This can manifest itself as an orgy, where a group shares indiscriminate sex play—or hones in on one lucky person who is the focus of all that sexual attention. Group sex is generally found at sex parties—gatherings where sex is formally acknowledged by the hosts and attendees as the primary reason for the event. Sex parties can be held privately among a group of friends or hosted by clubs and organizations, and they range from homegrown affairs to the outrageous big-budget productions of swingers' organizations. Read more about swingers and sex parties in Chapter 8, "Public Sex."

Jealousy

Jealousy is the main issue (apart from safer-sex considerations) that couples face when experimenting with threesomes and more, and it's the first thing you need to think about before attempting a group tryst. Even couples who have established trust over time and are deeply committed to each other encounter jealousy from time to time, often unexpectedly. So it's no great leap of logic to assume that sharing something as intimate as your private, coupled sex life with another person—possibly a total stranger—might cause a flash of anger, a sense of being left out, or a feeling of betrayal. It's even more confusing when these feelings all happen at once, confounding your rosy expectations.

Think everything through and discuss your fears with your lover before you try a threesome. Think about exactly what it is you want to do in your fantasy scenario, what you don't want to do, and explore possibilities of what might happen that would upset you. Talk to your lover and find out his or her concerns and perspectives as well. Don't worry that talking about it beforehand will dampen the excitement of trying the fantasy in real life—

believe me, the conversation won't compare to the real-life threesome.

What are your boundaries for having sex with others? Will this be something you do only in each other's presence? Or are you interested in starting an "open relationship"? Polyamory, in its many varied and wonderful combinations, is another subject altogether, and there are a number of books and online resources on the subject. (See Chapter 13, "Resources.")

Many couples make rules for their adventures with others, setting limits intended to keep both partners comfortable with the shared sex play. For instance, a woman might feel okay with a sexual encounter that includes another woman and her boyfriend, but may want to set limits such as "no kissing," "no penis–vagina penetration," or "no oral sex." Others might make rules like "penetration is okay only if you're kissing me," "stay focused on me," "you can only touch him if you follow my instructions," or "only touch both of us at the same time." Imagine your partner kissing another lover, and if it makes you uncomfortable, take it off the menu. Your comfort level around particular sex acts will change over time, so don't feel that your rules are set in stone. You establish them for your partner—and your partnership—but you can change them if you feel good about the changes.

Don't emphasize your prohibitions, of course. Remember, also, to think about what might turn you on—and put that on the menu. Would you like your partner to watch you kiss, perform oral sex, or make love with a woman or a man? Perhaps you'd like to watch your lover doing the same things—better yet, watch your sweetie perform a sex act that really turns you on while you embrace the sexy stranger. Or perhaps you have a fantasy sex position in mind, where you're in the middle of a "love sandwich," giving and receiving in a daisy chain of oral sex. Strap-ons can make simultaneous penetrations come true in ways you've only imagined.

This is the cardinal rule for sex with extra partners: Do only the things that turn you on, make you hot, and make you both feel good. Your partnership should always be more important at every moment than the experience you're having. Don't be afraid to say that you can't deal with something, and don't be afraid to stop the action if you become upset. Check in with each other's feelings as often as possible. Remember, this is about a fantasy you share—if one of you is having a bad time, it's not working and should be changed or stopped. Many couples who successfully play with others make this a hard and fast rule: If one of them wants the experience to change in any way or to stop, it does.

Some couples have a "safe word," a word not commonly used in conversation which signals that one partner's limits have been reached. For instance, you can agree to use stoplight terminology: Green means "I'm good," yellow means "I'm uneasy" or "let's slow down," and red means "stop."

If your sweetie becomes upset, he or she is your first priority. If your partner calls code yellow, asks you to stop, or worse, leaves the room, drop everything and go to their emotional rescue. Jealousy is often uncontrollable and inexplicable, and it's vital that you not question you partner's judgment or feelings on this matter. They're possibly at their most hurt and vulnerable right now; there will be time later for a constructive conversation about what went wrong. Listen to them, do what you can to make them feel understood, and follow their instructions about what to do next. If your partner doesn't know what he or she wants, then it's time to switch activities altogether—get a beverage, take a time out, leave the room together. Don't make a show of apologizing to your guest—this will make your lover feel worse. Instead, inquire how your guest is feeling and then say you are going to take a break.

What if you're the one who's upset? Of course, if any part of the fantasy upsets you in the first place, you should not even attempt it. But if you were excited by the idea to begin with, but once the action starts, find yourself feeling jealous, left out, abandoned, uneasy, or angry—say so. Out loud. If you have a safe word, use it—immediately. Don't wait to see if your feelings get worse, and don't worry about what your lover and your guest will think of you. They'll likely be glad you said something when you did, and your partner will have a chance to be there when you need him the most. Don't feel guilty about spoiling a good time—if it was truly a good time you wouldn't have felt troubled. Stopping the activity is okay. You may feel that seeing your lover kiss another woman is too much for you, or that trying a three-some at all was a bad idea. You'll have opportunities for great sexual adventures throughout your relationship: This is just one of many you'll have together.

Jealously can be like a storm that rages in and quickly subsides. If you feel comfortable later, explore your feelings about what happened. Loss and powerless-ness are the main components of jealousy, and something you saw probably triggered the primal fear of losing your lover to another person. It hurts, it feels like betrayal, and it calls into question your trust in your partner. Were you feeling in danger of losing your sweetie, or was it the feeling of exclusion that triggered you? Did you feel like you needed to compete? Were you not feeling good about yourself in general? Take these questions to your lover, even if you don't have the answers for yourself. Talk about what you felt, what happened, and give your partner a chance to tell you how he or she feels about the situation and your concerns. Decide whether your feelings are strong enough to change your mind about experimenting with threesomes. If you both want to continue playing with the fantasy, ask your lover to help you come up with solutions, rules, or limits for handling any negative feelings that might come up again.

Adding Someone New

So you've fantasized about it, given it serious thought, and talked it over with your lover—now what? You know you want it—now you just have to get it!

In your conversations about multiple-partner fantasies, talk about your ideal types and meeting scenarios. Discuss what qualities (like gender, looks, body type, sexual experience) attract you in order to clarify who you're looking for. Make an agreement that you'll only play with someone whom you're both attracted to. Be flexible with your partner's ideas of what is attractive, and also with what you'll find acceptable in reality. We all have a fantasy fuck in mind, but everyone knows that what happens in real life is usually quite different from what we'd imagined. And this is almost always a good thing.

Finding a suitable new partner may seem difficult, but you'll probably be surprised at how many prospects you find once you start looking. A surprising number of individuals out there prefer the safety, boundaries, and established trust that a tryst with a couple can provide. And the people you're looking for will be looking for you, too.

You may already have someone—or a few some-ones—in mind for your erotic adventure; you might be looking for the experience of a threesome with no one in particular; or your fantasy might be about trying your luck with strangers. Your options are open: The possibil-ities include approaching someone you know, going out to clubs or bars on sexually themed nights, attending sex parties or swingers' functions, and yes, advertising.

Friends and acquaintances might seem appealing as potential sex partners, but there is a lot to consider before you approach someone you know. The risks are obvious—rejection, loss of friendship, or a lot of discom-fort if the person is a coworker or a regular companion. Consider as off limits anyone whose workplace you fre-quent, such as your local coffee shop, unless you already have an amorous outside-of-work relationship blooming, and everyone is clear about boundaries. As with any sexual relationship, you stand to lose someone as a friend if the proposal, or the suggestion of one, isn't well received. Or if the experience proves less than satisfying.

If you do decide to pursue someone you know, look for clues that would indicate an interest in your fantasy. Ask yourself if your acquaintance is sexually adventur-ous—think about whether they are comfortable talking to you openly about sex and whether they have ever mentioned your particular fantasy. But even if you know they're into trying a threesome, it may still be beyond the boundaries of your friendship to propose such a fun-damental change to its parameters. Find out. Tell him or her what you and your lover are interested in, and see how they react. If the response is positive, be direct. Tell them that there's no pressure—they aren't to answer you right away, and you'd like to discuss it again if they feel comfortable.

Directness can be scary at first, but it's your most helpful tool. Being honest about your fantasies, expectations, concerns, and boundaries is your insurance against miscommunication, mistrust, and mishaps. And it can keep you from getting involved with someone incompatible. But most important of all, articulating what you want is the best way to make your fantasies come true, especially with sexual scenarios and when dealing with strangers.

Couples who cruise together might want to create a private code for communicating to each other their interest in a new candidate they are "interviewing," in order to avoid the embarrassment of giving mixed signals. The question "Are you thirsty?" could be your code for "What do you think of this guy?" A no would mean "no way," and a yes would give the go-ahead to flirt and play. It's a very good idea to have another code that means, "Let's move on" or "Get me outta here."

Negotiating your desires can be a matter of a quick conversation over drinks, or can take days or weeks of getting to know each other. There might be a lot to discuss, such as fantasy details, rules and limits, safe words, what type of sex is okay, safer sex (who's got condoms), spending the night or the weekend together, who pays for the whipped cream or the hotel room, and so on. You'll talk about all of this as the planning progresses, and everyone has the option of changing their minds as the actual event unfolds. Granted, negotiation can be as simple as "My boyfriend and I think you're really hot, and we have a room upstairs if you're interested." But you'll have more time for fun, for relaxing, and getting into the action if you get certain details out of the way—and out into the open—first. Play parties and sex parties have conduct rules for approaching potential sex partners—don't try anything until you're clear on the rules, and consult your hosts if you have questions.

First Impressions

The potential partners you and your sweetie set your sights on will bring their own desires, lusts, expectations, and limits to the experience, just as you will. Listen, ask questions, and check in with them whenever it seems appropriate.

When you make your approach, be keenly aware of what you're presenting—remember that first impressions are everything here. If one of you has elected to do the talking, be sure that you don't do *all* the talking, because you want your potential playmate to know you and your partner are equally interested. Otherwise, they might wonder whose idea this was anyway. Making the approach as a couple is ideal. Or, if you're in a male-female partnership, try approaching together. Having the woman make the approach as a way to assure the new prospect that it's her idea, might work well—but be aware that this can also come off as creepy. No one wants to go home with a couple in which one partner has been "put up to it" and the other partner's intentions (especially the guy's) are unclear. A woman, for instance, will be very reluctant to go upstairs with you and your boyfriend if she thinks you've been put out as "bait" for an upcoming and possibly unwelcome switch.

Just as you should never touch anyone without asking permission first, don't make any assumptions about the individual(s) you invite into your sex lives. They need not only equal affection (and orgasms!), but also extra consideration for the range of emotions they may experience. Don't allow them to feel left out, and do be aware of what they want from you. If they're cold toward you but hot for your lover, don't go any further, and if you sense any indifference or ambivalence toward your partnership, your boundaries, or your feelings, it's time to move on.

Get Together, and Get Off

You've talked, you've searched, and you've found your new partner—now it's playtime. Try these suggestions:

- Smile and laugh as much as possible. Nothing's sexier, more relaxing, or warmer than humor and confidence. Be silly, have fun, and be a big flirt.
- Break the ice physically by playing a sexy game, trading massages, watching porn, reading a sexy story aloud, taking a shower or hot tub—or be bold and just start taking off your clothes.
- Play with the balance of power. Elect one person to direct the action, or take turns being in charge.
- Always wear sexy underwear.
- Bring sex toys. Vibrators can keep your arousal level high when you're not being directly stimulated. Or you can masturbate with your trusty Hitachi while watching the others. A butt plug can be set in place for hands-free anal stimulation, and there are arrays of vibrators available that can be worn like panties, some even operated by remote control. Just be sure to follow cleanliness guidelines for sharing toys.
- Dildos and harnesses can make a threesome seem like an orgy. They can be used by women and men alike.
- Always have a stock of safer-sex supplies. Lube, condoms (latex and nonlatex), gloves, finger cots, and

dental dams should be in your fun stash. Make birth-control decisions well in advance.

- Always, always, always bring lube. Even if you think you don't need it, you should be using it anyway, for both pleasure and safety. Slicked-up parts feel wonderful, and natural lubrication isn't always reliable. Use a lube that's water-based, unflavored, uncolored, and doesn't contain added sugars or glycerin. Why? Because these additives contribute to yeast infections in women—not a nice memento of your encounter.
- Try a lightly kinky prop such as a blindfold and feathers. Don't use the blindfold on the newcomer unless they explicitly ask.
- Bring out the really kinky props. If everyone involved is consenting and is well versed in S/M practices, the many delightful enhancements and accoutrements of S/M can have the effect of pouring gasoline on your threesome's fire. Punishments such as paddling and whipping have gravity with extra people as witnesses, helpers, or additional naughty girls or boys.
- Role-playing becomes more realistic—and more arousing—with another person playing along. For instance, a doctor and nurse can attend to a patient's every need, or two male police officers can barter for trade with a lady who "just can't get another ticket."

Sex Positions

You can do a lot with several bodies, and the potential for pleasure is limitless. Here are some ideas for a threesome:

- Team up and perform oral sex together on the hapless third partner.

- Use your hands to masturbate one partner while another licks your genitals.
- Hold your partner on your lap (facing outward), with your legs spread, while your play partner performs oral sex on one or both of you.
- One partner lies on their back while the second sits on their face and the third licks or fucks their genitals.
- Put the lucky newcomer on all fours while you lick or penetrate their genitals and your partner enjoys their mouth.
- Make a "sandwich" out of someone by putting him or her in the middle. A man in the middle can penetrate one partner while being penetrated by the other's fingers, penis, or dildo. A woman in the middle can be penetrated while penetrating another with her strap-on.
- One partner can fuck another with a strap-on while the third performs oral sex on—either!
- Lick each other's genitals or give fellatio in a "daisy chain" of oral sex.

Hooking Up: Cruising and Advertising

Some couples get lucky and discover a playmate right in their own backyard and have their fun without having to search. They might meet someone unexpectedly, at a café or party, or just open a new door with an old friend. But most of us aren't that lucky. We have to work at it a bit—which is fine, because as any couple knows, a little work and patience always pays off, especially when it comes to sex. If any of the following ideas sounds appealing to you, visit the Resources chapter for further study.

One option is to "cruise" for your new companion—that is, pick someone up in a bar, club, or other known pickup spot. The benefits of the quick pickup are many: You have a variety of prospects to choose from; you get as many chances to hook up as the number of people you feel like talking to; there is a greater chance for anonymous encounters (especially if you travel away from home); and one-night stands or quick-and-dirty encounters are always the special of the day.

If this sounds like your cup of tea, do some research to find out where evenings for singles, bisexuals, or social events with sexual themes occur in your town. Check the weekly newspapers in the nearest major city for sexy events such as fetish parties, erotic dance contests, or even adult Halloween parties. Make sure the place you decide on is for adults only and has a sexual theme of interest to you on the night you go to increase your chances of finding someone compatible. Swingers' and sex parties are terrific places for finding new people to add to your twosome—you can read more about them in Chapter 8, "Public Sex." You can also check out hotels and bed-and-breakfast retreats that openly advertise or acknowledge sexual activity among guests.

Some couples know exactly what they want, and if that's you, placing an ad is probably the best way to get it. All major metropolitan areas have weekly newspapers (or their online versions): The back pages are where you'll find the sexual ads. These are great for finding people who are looking for what you've got, or for advertising your wishes for someone out there to grant. There will be a section for couples, possibly with subcategories; read the ads thoroughly to see what will work best for your situation. You can advertise online as well, but to find someone local you'll need to use local resources (including online bulletin boards and personal ad services). If you don't care where your partners are located, or want to have cybersex threesomes with cameras and streaming video, you can place your ad in whatever venue you feel is appropriate.

Read other people's ads to get an idea of how to write yours and be as clear and concise as you can. Keep in mind that people can be pretty dishonest in their ads, so answer ads with caution. And be aware that ads asking for "generosity" or "donations" are code for sex workers. If you feel that advertising, sex parties, and cruising aren't your game and you'd prefer a more straightforward arrangement, you might consider hiring a sex worker or two to fulfill your fantasies. If so, read Chapter 7, "Strip Clubs, Phone Sex, and Call Girls—for Two."

California Dreaming

BY ALISON TYLER

Alden wanted to watch another man fuck me.

You just can't say it any plainer than that.

As he rolled me over in bed, parting my long legs and sliding his cock deep inside me, he whispered his favorite fantasy. "Just once," he assured me. "Oh, baby. Just one time. I know what you're like in bed. I know how you feel, and how you look, and how you taste. But I want to watch another man learn those sexy secrets. I want to see you come while he takes care of you."

"He?" I asked.

Doggie-style lets Alden go in deep, and for a moment, he couldn't respond. But even though I was as turned on as my man, I wouldn't let up, waiting only a moment before murmuring more insistently, *"He?"* as I gazed into the mirror above our bed and stared at our reflections. Alden is dark-haired and bronze-skinned, with gray-green eyes that sheen with an insatiable sexual appetite.

"You know who—" Alden said, slamming faster now, really fucking me. I slid one hand between my legs and touched my clit, fingering myself gently as Alden continued, "you *know*, baby. The pool guy."

Oh, god. The pool guy.

Alden and I rent a large, Spanish-style bungalow in sun-drenched Santa Monica. The best part about the house is the backyard pool—a lush aqua gem in a lagoon setting. And the best part about the pool is the stunning man who comes once a week to clean it. Talk about your California dreaming.... Will is tall and long-limbed, with birch-blond hair and eyes that rival the blue of the deep end of our oval pool. When I first saw him, I felt that naughty pang you get when you're in a long-term relationship and notice a particularly beautiful specimen.

Although I've never been much of a swimmer, I instantly began to fantasize about taking a decadent dip into the pleasurable waters of sex with Will. Now that I'd been given free reign to enjoy these fantasies, they came more and more often. In bed, in the shower, in line at the grocery store. Whenever I closed my eyes, that vision awaited me. I was California daydreaming, in a constant state of enhanced arousal. Somehow, though, the naughtiness didn't disappear even though these fantasies were green-lighted by my man. Because Alden wasn't suggesting a threesome, where he might go out and have a beer with Will at the tapas bar around the corner, explain the sex-charged situation, then casually invite him into our boudoir—no, he wanted to watch, surreptitiously watch, while I got it on with the pool guy.

And the thing of it is, nothing had ever excited me more.

"Here's the deal," I explained to my boyfriend after many pleasurable fantasy sessions. "I don't want to plan this to death. If it happens, it happens; otherwise, we can forget about it. This isn't something I'm willing to force."

That was good enough for Alden—and as it turned out, he didn't have to wait long. Next week, when Will arrived, I knew what to do. I walked by the pool in my indecently short white robe and settled myself on one of the outdoor wood-and-canvas lounges, as if I were innocently positioned there to catch a few mid-afternoon rays. Alden was upstairs in his office, and I knew that if he looked out through the blinds he'd be able to see everything.

"Hey," Will said to me, quickly glancing up from his job.

"Hey," I said back, untying my white terry-cloth robe and letting it fall open. I wasn't wearing anything underneath. Not a string bikini. Not a skimpy thong. With my shades on, I pretended to completely ignore Will, but I knew he wasn't able to do the same with me. No straight man could have. His eyes were focused on the silky expanse of skin showing in the parting of the robe. I could almost feel him grow hard from where he stood.

After a few minutes, he walked to my side of the pool, then to my side of the lounge, and finally he sat down right at the edge.

"You're going to burn," he said, reaching for the suntan lotion.

"You mean it's going to get so hot?"

He looked at me, eyebrows raised.

"You know," I smiled, shaking the robe off completely. "When we fuck—"

That's all the encouragement he needed. But before we continued, I reached into the pocket of my robe for a condom.

"You're prepared," he grinned.

"Like you wouldn't believe."

"And what does Alden think about all this?" he asked, as he rolled on the condom.

"We have an arrangement..." I whispered.

"Oh," he breathed, "an *arrangement.*"

His hands were rich with the oil and he slid them up and down my naked body. I breathed in deep to catch the tropical scent of the oil mixed with the bougainvillea growing on the stucco and the sweet honeysuckle way at the back of the yard. I sighed and arched, and Will rolled me over and pressed me down on the towel, his shorts open, his body on mine.

I visualized Alden watching every move. I could see it in my mind as he pressed himself up to the blinds, one firm hand on his rigid cock, tugging as he watched Will enter me from behind. That thought brought me even higher as Will gripped my auburn ponytail and steeled me for what turned out to be a wild ride. His rock-hard body slammed into mine with each thrust. The combination of the action and the thought of my man watching everything had me slippery wet, with juices dripping down my inner thighs.

"God, you're hot," Will sighed as he bucked against me.

"On fire—" I agreed, pushing back into him, meeting and matching him stride for stride. I didn't look up to the second floor as I came. I closed my eyes and let the world disappear. Will brought his fingertips to my swollen clit, extending the pleasure for me as he drove in deep.

"Where is he?" Will hissed against my neck. "Where?"

"Upstairs."

Will jutted his chin upward, and I felt a connection made between the three of us: me, Alden, and my new lover. Or should I say, "our" new lover.

"Tell him to come downstairs," Will demanded.

"You—" I told him, sighing. "Oh, Will, you do it."

He called out Alden's name, and then I heard the sound of feet on the steps, and the screen door opening. I looked up to see my man standing there, a waiting, willing smile on his face.

California dreaming? Maybe. But every once in a while even the most fantastic dreams can come true.

6

Weaving a Spell: Striptease, Hot Talk, and Erotic Massage

Nothing weaves a spell of seduction like a sexy striptease or a sensuous lap dance. You can bring a lover to full arousal—and some even to orgasm—with dirty talk. A rousing bout of phone sex can leave you both hot for round two in person. And a surprise erotic massage can turn therapeutic touch into an incendiary encounter. Each of these skills has been honed by the pros: exotic dancers, phone-sex workers, and erotic masseuses. When you bring these skills home, your lover will think they've found an erotic genie in a bottle, and you'll reap the rewards of feeling like the sexiest vixen alive.

Putting your sexuality onstage, talking a blue streak, and rubbing 'em down might seem daunting at first— but these skills of seduction and sex play can make you as compelling as a force of nature. Confidence and sexiness are the seductive powers of both the virile player and the femme fatale, and when you develop these deceptively simple talents, you won't have to be an exhibitionist or have a dancer's body to make it happen. All you need is the desire to light his or her fire, and to learn a few tricks that'll turn it into a roaring blaze. Your goal is an encounter that turns you both on.

Confidence

Every day, tens of thousands of women (and men) get up on stage (or in front of the camera) and take off their clothes. And most of them look damn sexy doing it, too, peeling off their panties with style, stroking their bodies proudly and with grace. But behind every sure step, every inviting gyration, is the person who at one point had to get up the guts to do it. Unlike Hollywood stars, these folks usually don't look "perfect," but they do look like screamingly desirable sex kittens and tomcats. Now, you're not exactly getting ready to perform for a roomful of strangers (though if you are, yay!). You are probably interested in putting on an erotic show for someone who matters very much—or at least whom you want to wow enough to get into their pants. So, you have to wonder, how the heck did all those strippers get themselves up onto that stage? What can you learn from the pros that will help you perform your own wickedly sexy seduction?

First of all, professional strippers have learned to accept what they've got. Because we only see a narrow range of beauty in our media, we forget that everyone has the same complaints about themselves. Most people don't look like packaged porn stars or Hollywood stars in real life. Come to think of it, most of those porn stars and Hollywood types look a bit odd in real life. Erotic performers have learned to let go of their inner critics, for at least a few songs anyway, and let their sexy moves and their careful attention to appearance speak for them. Time and time again, it works, simply because confidence and sexiness are riveting.

Think about what bothers you. Chances are high your concerns boil down to a few very common anxieties:

I'm worried that I'll look ridiculous.

Plan your scene, learn your moves, try on your outfits, and test any makeup ahead of time. If you've done your planning, the only thing your audience will see is a sexy someone making their fantasies come true. They'll also be excited that you went to so much effort just for them—not many people do. The only thing that might show is your nervousness, but that will disappear after the first few minutes.

What if I screw it up?

Make your routine or seduction "idiot proof" by going over it step by step, repeatedly, and don't leave anything to the last minute. Take every precaution to remove distractions, from turning off your phone to securing pets that might suddenly appear underfoot. If you're klutzy, be prepared to laugh, smile wickedly at your prey, and distract them by cranking the heat of your moves up a notch. A sense of humor combined with erotic purpose and determination will make them forget all about the spilled drink—especially if you lick it off their hands, face, or neck. Plus, ripped stockings are quite sexy.

My body isn't what I want it to be.

Join the biggest club in the world. Everyone feels this way on one level or another, even the "perfect" people. If you don't like it, make a plan to change it. If you can't change it, work it. Make the most of what you've got. Chances are high that you're a lot sexier than you think, because sexiness comes from inside, not the outside. If you're worried about "stacking up" to others with the size of your breasts or the size of your basket, or other measurement concerns, remember that bigger boobs (or a bigger bulge) won't make you sexier—they'll just make you someone with big boobs (or a big basket). And yes, people can be insensitive critics and say inappropriate things—but if you find yourself performing for someone like this, never perform for that person again.

Preparations

You'll need to decide on the basic elements that create atmosphere, character, and an aura of sexiness. First, choose your persona, the personality that you want to project in your performance. Then decide on your outfit, music, lighting, the time and date, and a fitting location for it all to take place. Watch how-to videos on erotic dancing, or even TV movie depictions of erotic performers to get ideas for moves and routines.

Begin planning at least a week in advance. Give yourself plenty of time to create a routine, learn your moves, shop for clothing and props, and take care of any miscellaneous details. Don't wait until the last minute to arrange childcare or send your roommates to the movies; you'll want your house empty, with no chance of unwanted interruptions, so take care of this well ahead of time. Also make a checklist for turning off your phone, and closing windows, curtains, or doors for maximum privacy. Give your lover a little advance warning. You want to surprise your sweetie in a good way, not catch them off guard at the wrong time. Make a date with them for a romantic evening—you don't have to let on what's going to happen, just that they're in for a sexy surprise.

Pick a persona—and dress the part. Of course, you could always be yourself, but donning a character can give you lots of room to play with your props, costuming, makeup, music, and your routine. Just as a French maid or police officer can arouse and excite, your sex-kitten self can set the night on fire with a sensual outfit and slinky lingerie. Just ensure that whatever you wear makes you feel sexy, and give consideration to how you'll be slipping out of it. Skirts are usually easier than pants, and smoothly pulling a shirt or dress off over your head may require some practice. (Though male strippers do manage to show off their chests while removing neckties, business shirts, and even three-piece suits.) If you want to wear pasties—little sequined or tasseled patches on the nipples—buy them along with professional pastie glue at strippers' outlets; don't try to make them at home.

Atmosphere and setting provide the finishing touches. Decide where you want to slither and shake. Bedrooms are nice, but also consider the kitchen, dining room, garage, and bathroom—or farther afield, like a hotel room. If you are playing a persona, pick a location that suits your role—for example, a mechanic in the garage, a cowgirl in the barn, or a waitress in the dining room. Lighting should be low but not dark, and you can add effect with focused halogens or colored bulbs. Test the look of your room at the same time of day or night as your planned performance. Choose your music, then make a playlist, or burn a CD of

MP3s, adding slower songs at the end of your routine to prolong the romantic atmosphere. Make sure there is a comfortable chair for your lucky audience member, and enough room for you to wiggle, gyrate, and strip for the "front row."

How to Strip

Let the games begin! Learn a few steps and dance moves, create a routine, and then practice, practice, practice. I recommend choosing two or three songs to plan a routine around, songs that make you feel sexy, with a rhythm that you can slither, shimmy, shake, and grind along with. After all, you'll be dancing to the music—just any old song will not do.

Remember throughout your routine to hold your head high, keep your chest out, your shoulders back, and your back arched. This is how strippers and models emphasize their best features. This, and a lot of attitude.

Visualize an image or scenario that makes you feel like the queen or king of the world. Everyone who's performed erotically has a visualization that gets them in the right frame of mind. One dancer I interviewed, from the legendary Mitchell Brothers' O'Farrell Theater in San Francisco, told me, "I just imagine the money going into my g-string, and it just keeps getting filled. Then I'm taking the money into the bank, and I'm so rich they take me into the vault, which is full of my money. Sometimes I'm on the red carpet at a Hollywood premiere, with hundreds of fans and photos being taken. Other times I'm accepting an Academy Award." Think of your most glamorous fantasy, where you're irresistibly beautiful, and make it as detailed and vivid as possible. Then pretend you're there, and start your routine.

You have to learn to walk before you can fly, and erotic dancing is no exception: Your first move is to learn how to strut. Your walk will be the foundation for every move you make. Begin by placing your feet as if you were following an imaginary straight line. Exaggerate your hips by giving each step a sideways swing before landing on your line. Practice walking with your hands on your hips, on top of your head, at the back of your neck, and beneath your breasts. While walking, you can play with your breasts, run your hands seductively all over your butt, hips, and torso, muss up your hair, or do anything else that shows you off to best effect and tells your audience where to look. To turn right, start with your right foot forward, draw a half-circle to the right, and pivot heel-to-toe. Try it, and you'll see what I mean.

When you're not strutting, you'll have an arsenal of moves for stopping, pivoting, changing direction, and taking off your clothes. For women, your hips are your sexiest weapons. For men, it's the pelvis which can roll and grind. Practice rolling your hips, or grinding your pelvis, in circles at slow, medium, and fast speeds, then simultaneously with your hands in motion, touching your body seductively or slowly peeling off clothing. Grind your hips forward and back at different speeds as well, and remember to display your hip moves from all angles: front, sides, and back. Move your hips or pelvis in figure eights for the full effect; this move looks especially good from behind, when you're bent slightly at the waist with an arched back. In general, it's easiest to do your hip moves with your feet staggered. Rely on your hip moves if you lose your place in your routine.

Intermittently caress your entire body from head to toe throughout your routine. Practice long, languorous strokes with your hands while standing with your back to your audience, in a kneeling position (stroking from knees to your hair), and on the floor (on your back, giving a sideways view). You should especially concentrate on touching and feeling your breasts (or chest), which may feel a little strange at first but is essential to your seduction. Play with your breasts, knead and rub them (guys, go for your pecs and abs), close your eyes and show your lover just how good it feels. Imagine that your breasts are being touched for the first time. Get into it!

Your moves should be serpentine and erotic. Slow down your movements, more than you think you should, and pepper your routine with touching, bending, and removing articles of clothing. Make as much eye contact as possible, except when you get carried away in the rapture of touching yourself. Only turn your back to your partner if you want to show your hip moves or open your shirt. Remember, it's all about teasing, making your partner long to see your naked body. Remove your shirt first, then your skirt, bra, and panties (assuming this is your costume), in that order.

Take your time removing each article of clothing. Consider leaving your shoes, hat, or garters on. Tease your audience by offering small glimpses of what's to come. Try unbuttoning a shirt with a hip or pelvic move for each button, pause to stroke your breasts or chest, unbutton all the way, and then let the shirt slowly slide from your arms to the floor, all the while moving your hips or grinding your pelvis. Always gently brush clothing out of the way with your feet.

Pants are tough to remove gracefully. Play with the zipper or buttons. Turn your back and play peek-a-boo with your butt. Bend over and look at your audience upside down through your legs. Get down on the floor, roll onto your stomach, and slither out of your pants as you get up.

Once you have practiced taking off your clothes and learned a few dance steps, make a plan for your routine. Here are some moves you can incorporate into your own routine:

- Arrange your scene so that you can come in from a side entrance. Strut to center "stage," pivot, and face your prey.
- Rotate your hips, moving your hands over your body. Stop, roll your hips in a figure eight, and massage your breasts (or work your pecs).
- Pivot until you're facing away from your subject and slide your hands from breasts to toes, smiling from between your legs.
- Strut, turn, hold position, and move hips or pelvis.
- As you begin to unbutton your top, slowly rotate your hips or grind your pelvis. Open the buttons in synch with your hips. With your shirt open, walk toward your lover with hands on hips and then resume fondling your breasts (or chest). Slowly writhe out of your shirt.
- Remember that your hands become your lover's eyes and wishes. Touch yourself everywhere you think they're aching to touch you.
- Toy with your lover by getting closer and closer during your routine. On your first approach, touch your prey. Stand right between their legs, gently uncrossing and opening them if necessary. You decide when it's okay for your partner to touch you—often, it's more fun to make them wait, and you can gently return their roving hands to their knees so they know who's in charge.

Lap Dance 101

When a striptease becomes a lap dance, you're dancing, removing clothing, and rubbing your body all over your lover. A lap dance is a glorified, sexified dry hump put to music—but when it is between lovers it is far hotter and more intimate than any description.

Here are some good moves to try:

- Use your full body to stroke your partner, moving from their knees slowly up their thighs, hips, waist, and chest, stopping at the shoulders.
- Mess up their hair.
- Move your breasts from eye level onto the chest, then slide them down to crotch level. Your hands can follow their path and steady you as you sink to your knees.
- Caress your breasts and make sultry eye contact.
- Work bits and pieces of a striptease into your lap dance.
- Play with your hair, or any props you might have— for example, a maid might dust her audience from head to toe.
- Place one foot on their thigh (beware of high heels) and rotate your hips.
- Turn around to grind your butt into their crotch. Then lie back and press your whole body onto theirs, reaching back to play with their hair.
- Rub your breasts in their face.
- Straddle their legs and play with yourself.
- Grind your crotch onto their thigh.

Finish the routine any way you like—but the best way is with a hot bout of sex. From the start, your happy subject will be transfixed by your erotic show, and will have to make an effort to keep themselves from grabbing you, removing your clothes, and ravishing you on the spot. That's the point—get him or her as worked up as possible, but withhold sexual contact until you say so. If you choose to incorporate lap dancing with your strip routine, you'll be cranking up the heat every time you rub your body and breasts over their torso, tease by moving away, and then return for more. Pay special attention to grinding on the crotch area and, with a man, increasingly brushing up against his erection as you near the end of your show. For a finish, you can do any of the following:

- Take your partner's clothes off, too. Slowly peel off their shirt and open the top button of their pants, all the while continuing with your dancing and hip rotations.
- Slide down their body and remain on your knees to perform oral sex.
- Facing away, have sex in the "reverse cowgirl" position. Or turn around and ride him in the chair.
- Take your sweetie by the hand and lead them to the bedroom.
- Sink down to a kneeling position and pull your partner onto the floor with you.

The Art of Dirty Talk

Quiet, focused sex can be intense and climactic—but opening your mouth and telling your partner what you're thinking can really crank up the heat. Dirty talk makes hot sex even hotter and can come in handy when you're separated by distance but connected by a phone or DSL line.

Hot talk means simply giving your partner an explicit description of sex, in as much detail as possible, with some drama and good timing and carefully chosen words. You don't necessarily have to use vulgar language, and you never have to use terms you're uncomfortable with. On the flip side, if you generally don't use coarse words like "pussy" or "cock," hearing these words coming out of your mouth in a heated moment might just send your lover over the edge.

You can talk dirty before sex, during foreplay, or throughout the day in a series of phone messages or strategically placed notes. You can describe a sexual fantasy—yours or your partner's—in explicit detail from start to finish. Or, once you hit the sheets, you can describe what's actually happening right then and there. Further, you can tell your lover what you'd like them them to do, or what you'd like to do to them.

It's important to be as descriptive as possible. Slow down; don't rush anything. If you're concerned about saying dirty things out loud because it's new for you, find some private time, make a list of words you might have trouble with, and say them—out loud, over and over. Do it in front of a mirror. You may laugh at first— and it's even okay to laugh when you try it with your partner. What matters is that you speak the words and that your desire to turn yourself and your partner on says you *mean* it. If you still think it sounds silly, don't worry—when you say your words to your lover in person, it'll sound plenty sexy. Carol Queen, in *Exhibitionism for the Shy*, recommends talking dirty to yourself while you masturbate, using your arousal to help you get comfortable saying filthy things.

Find your sexiest voice. Some people have a difficult time hearing their own voice and might find that trying a few vocal exercises gives them a sexier and more resonant sound. Practice speaking not from your throat, but from the center of your chest, powering the air up from your belly. You can relax your face by stretching the muscles of your jaw, lips, and tongue. This will also improve your sound.

Speak softly by lowering the volume and the pitch. Try a sentence in a low whisper, deeper than your normal voice. Then try it louder and still deeper. Next, hum, keeping your mouth closed. Now speak the sentence in your low whisper, but with the same resonance as the hum. You'll use these different techniques to find the sexy voice that works best for you (and to gauge your volume over any background music). During sex, you'll be speaking in an unrushed tempo in your sexy, low voice. Ask your partner a few questions, and match their response in timing, volume, and urgency. You'll tune right into their arousal.

But what do you say during dirty talk? Because hot talk relies on your own creativity, figuring out what to say can be daunting. Describing a fantasy—which takes guts and a sense of adventure—is one of the simplest and most delicious ways to spice up sex. If you don't know where to start, let someone else provide the words—pick up an erotic short-story collection that focuses on fantasies for couples and borrow a fantasy. Read erotica, look for dirty stories online, and make a note of whatever turns you on.

Another trick is to describe what you're doing at the moment, but make it dirtier. For instance, if you're caressing his thigh, you can say: "Your thigh feels really good under my hand. I love touching you so close to your delicious cock. I can see you getting hard. Do you want me to touch your cock? I'd love to stroke you up and down your shaft, rub and press against your hard dick. It would feel so good to fondle your balls, slide my hand around the base of your shaft, and give it a squeeze. Then I could slide up your shaft and grip the tip of your cock in my soft fist." Get the idea? Then deliver on your promise, describing what you're doing every step of the way.

Once you unleash your dirty-talk skills, and what they can do for your sex life, you'll feel as if you've discovered a secret superhero power. Use your power to turn your good-girl persona into a tigress between the sheets, or your femme fatale identity into a prowling seductress. Dirty-talk skills can be used in bed, over the phone, in a chat room, in a crowded restaurant, or anywhere that turns you on. Mask, cape, and boots are optional.

Giving an Erotic Massage

No role-playing scenario involving nurses or masseuses can convince, no public hand job can really sing, no seductive pampering session can be complete without the tricks and delights of genital massage. Erotic massage is also a great skill if your fantasy is to sexually "service" your partner with your hands. I highly recommend watching the videos listed in the Resources chapter at the end of this book, especially those from The New School of Erotic Touch.

Plan your massage and meals accordingly; don't offer a massage to someone who has just eaten a large meal. If you have to eat, make it a light, sensual snack. Having your massage subject take a bath or shower beforehand is relaxing and warms up the skin. Have massage oil ready (unscented or lightly scented), some water-based lubricant for genital massage, and if you feel playful, other sensation toys such as feathers, fur mitts, or a soft body brush.

Before applying oil, slowly and sensually stroke your lover's entire body from head to toe with feathers, other sensation toys, or your caressing hands. Relax them with gentle strokes; try a variety of sensations on their skin to warm them up and awaken their senses. You may start with your lover on their stomach, giving a luxurious back-of-the-body massage before you roll them over and concentrate on the front. Or you can begin with the front for a more overtly sexual massage. Either way, don't start with the genitals (unless this is the plan and you know your partner is ready). Instead, tease, touch, and knead other areas such as the face, shoulders, back, chest, breasts, thighs, and hips. Really adventurous lovers can incorporate front-slide lap-dancing moves, essentially massaging with the whole body—an incredibly arousing experience for the recipient. Take time to work up your lover's arousal before you move to genital massage.

Oil is great for massage on external genitals but isn't latex-compatible (it will break condoms easily) and isn't suitable for vaginal penetration. Because oil is difficult to flush from the vaginal canal, it can remain there and encourage bacterial infections, so use water-based lube for vaginal penetration. Plan ahead if you use condoms during sex.

You can apply lube to your partner's genitals in a number of sexy ways. Pour it directly onto their penis or vulva from a height of a few inches or more; warm it in your hands first and smooth it on; or cup your hand over their genitals and pour the lube over the back of your hand, allowing it to seep through your fingers.

Massaging the Vulva

Try these tips for vulva massage:

- Cup your hand over her entire vulva and knead, rub in circles, or keep your hand still and apply pressure.
- Alternating hands, slide the lube downward, from the pubic bone to the lower part of the vulva. Reverse direction and pull the lube up.
- If you massage the anal area, don a latex or polyurethane glove. (Never allow anal bacteria to enter the vagina; it can cause infection.)
- Rub the outer lips in small circles with flattened fingers. Gently pull and tug on them in sync, using the thumb and forefinger of both hands.
- With one or two fingers, rub upward or downward along the inside of the outer lips, along the sides of the clitoris. Circle in the furrow for variation.
- Pay attention to her body language. If she seems to pull away, reduce your pressure. If she's grinding into your hand, follow her cues and match her rhythm.
- Ask her what she wants.
- Build up to massaging her clit. It will be extremely sensitive to direct touch, though less so as she becomes more aroused. Start with several flattened fingers to diffuse the sensation. Find a spot she likes on the side, top, or below the glans of her clit. Play around with sensations here, then find a rhythm and stick to it.
- She may or may not want penetration—ask. If she does, insert one or two fingers (more if she asks) and allow them to follow the natural curve of her vaginal canal. Keep your fingers firm, but follow her internal angle. Make your in-and-out rhythm steady and slow, quickening when she requests it.

- When you get a rhythm going that she likes, don't stop or change it.

Massaging the Penis

Try these strokes for the penis:

- Massage lube all over his cock and balls, and into the furrows where his thighs meet his body.
- Alternating hands, slide the lube downward, from the pubic bone to the top of his cock and balls. Reverse direction and pull the lube up.
- Using a glove for anal massage is highly recommended, though not necessary unless your hands or his penis will be in vaginal contact later.
- Alternating hands, circle the base of his shaft and pull the lube up to the top.
- The tip of his penis is usually the most sensitive part. Stimulating him here may be too intense, though this may change as he becomes more aroused.
- Include his testicles in your affections. Give them gentle squeezes and tugs, and roll lube over the surface.
- Hold the base of his cock in one hand and stroke the top with the other hand. The stroking hand can twist up, pull up, move up and down, or grip rhythmically in a fist.
- Hold the base of his cock and pull downward on his testicles.
- Begin a stroking rhythm on his shaft, using both hands to form a long tunnel, holding the base, or using one hand only on the end.

Erotic massage proceeds in stages of intensity, from rubbing lube onto your squirming sweetie all the way to intense and rhythmic strokes at the end. Begin with the lighter stuff. Vary your techniques until your partner's arousal really builds, then narrow your strokes to simple rhythmic ones, focusing on a single final technique to bring them to orgasm. Many people make the mistake of changing strokes and pacing as orgasm nears. Rather, help your lover concentrate by zeroing in on the technique that will take them over the edge.

The signs of impending orgasm will vary from person to person. For some, it will be obvious—they'll tell you! For others, you'll have to look for physiological signs. Increased breathing, perspiration, a rosy flush that spreads over the face, throat, and chest, and erect nipples (though not always) are good signs to look for. In most men, the cock will grow hard and the testicles will draw close to the body, though some men may not get hard at all, so you'll have to ask if you're not sure. Women will show fullness and firmness in their clit and outer labia, and some will get clit erections. Wetness isn't always a sure sign of arousal, so don't rely on it as a sign of impending orgasm.

When your lover starts to orgasm, keep doing whatever you are doing—don't stop until the orgasm subsides. If you're with a man who ejaculates (some men don't), decide where you want his come to go—in your hand, on his stomach, in your mouth, or elsewhere. The tip of his penis might become suddenly very sensitive right after orgasm, so don't continue stroking after he comes unless you know he likes it. The same goes for women: If she ejaculates, decide where you want to be when it happens. Stop stroking after she comes, because clits and G-spots can grow incredibly sensitive (in an almost painful way) right after orgasm—unless she instructs you to keep going. Conclude your massage with some sexy cleanup—a fresh towel is always nice, or you can slip away to the bathroom and prepare a warm washcloth. Finish by wrapping your partner in a blanket, snuggling up, and dining on pre-prepared snacks and revitalizing beverages.

7

Strip Clubs, Phone Sex, and Call Girls— For Two

Seeing a professional sex worker is often the easiest way for couples to add a third partner to their sex play, no strings attached. Phone sex, a visit to a strip club, or an hour at a peep show can be a safe way to test the waters before actually engaging in sex with a stranger. You can learn a lot from the pros in addition to learning more about yourselves, your likes and dislikes, and uncovering further fantasies for you both to share.

Perhaps you want to watch your sweetie get a lap dance from a beautiful stripper, or you want to watch your lover watching *you* get one. Strip joints and "gentlemen's clubs" can fill that fantasy. Call girls and prostitutes offer the possibility of a sexual encounter with a stranger whom you will never see again, making them perfect for trying a no-strings threesome, experimenting with girl–girl sex, or watching each other have sex with a stranger.

What's great about playing with pros is the anonymity, confidentiality, and convenience, not to mention the added plus of "ordering up" the specific sex acts you both want. It's like ordering a sumptuous meal and having it arrive hot and just the way you like it. You decide together what you want, and you ask for it—it's that simple. Sex workers have seen it all and will make no judgments about your interests. They are adept at knowing how to give you what you want, and will make it clear when it's not something they do. They are people who provide intimate services: They are in the business of making sexual fantasies come true.

Strip Clubs and Lap Dances

Couples venturing into strip clubs are much more prevalent than most people think. While the media depict topless bars, peep shows, and strip joints as populated by male patrons, with women in an entertainment capacity only, in reality that scenario has become dated as more and more women and couples join the audience. Groups of women, single women, and heterosexual couples provide an ever-growing customer base for erotic dancers, and they will often get as much attention from the performers as the guys at the next table. Many dancers are excited to perform for couples. If you and your partner bring paper bills and smiles, you'll both have a blast.

Before you both go rushing off to the Titty Twister Bar and Grill, give your adventure a little forethought. What are you hoping to get out of going to a strip club— your curiosity satisfied, a thrill, or something more?

Decide which partner will be the focus of attention for lap dances and who will do the tipping, because the one with the money will typically be the object of the flirting and erotic displays. Perhaps you both want a lap dance (from the same girl or from two at one time). How will you feel seeing your lover getting a lap dance from another woman? Patrons in American clubs are usually not allowed to touch the dancers, except to place money in their outfits—if that. Even with those restrictions, seeing your lover get a lap dance still might push your buttons. Don't let jealousy take you by surprise; be honest with yourself about what you are okay with seeing. If you're not sure, make an agreement to stop or go somewhere else if either of you begins to feel bad.

Exotic-dance establishments (another name for strip clubs) feature women in various states of undress dancing on stages. They often provide other varieties of erotic entertainment as well. Depending on the club and local laws, there may be lap dancing, where you are seated in a chair and the dancer rubs and grinds her body all over you. You pay by the song. (More about payment below.) Lap dancing can take place in the middle of the club, along special chairs against a back wall, or privately, in curtained-off rooms.

Some places may have private peep booths where dancers perform erotic acts like masturbation for you from behind glass. You pay by the minute as well as a separate charge per act. Some businesses have only peep booths; some have rooms where private booths face a small glass-enclosed stage on which one or more women will perform for you. (More on peep shows in the next section.) Other clubs have strippers onstage and table shows in separate rooms, or "private VIP rooms," where women perform with sex toys literally on your table, solo or in twos, and you can request the sex acts you desire. Quite a few higher-end clubs have given thought to the many ways they can get you to spend your money on the entertainment, and you'll likely come across more activities than those I've listed here.

Strip clubs are public establishments, usually bars, where the atmosphere is sexually supercharged but no sex happens on the premises. There are seedy clubs where anything goes, but you should be aware that these come with many risks. Depending on the state and county laws regarding nudity and alcohol, and how lax the individual strip club is willing to be, what you find in the clubs will vary. Some jurisdictions don't allow nudity in establishments that serve alcohol, and some allow partial nudity with alcohol. Others might condone booze, boobs, and even no panties, but the dancers must cover their nipples or they're considered indecent. It's perplexing. The bottom line is that you might have to forgo alcohol to see completely nude dancers or enjoy

How will they treat me at the strip club?

Although I interviewed many strippers and club patrons, and spoke to boy- and girlfriends of exotic dancers, nothing prepared me for the mixed reactions I got when I ventured into strip clubs as part of my "research." I found myself—young, female, sexily dressed, looking much like the dancers onstage—ignored by male patrons, who barely glanced at me while they fixated on the naked women. The dancers' reactions were all over the map, from avoiding eye contact, and physically avoiding me, to excitedly jumping in my lap, giving me more of a show (and more physical license) than they gave the men in the club. My boyfriend and I felt like the hottest couple alive. How will they treat you? Any, or all, of the above.

your drinks while topless-only hotties give you lap dances. In most of the U.S., lap dancers are clothed (creating interesting definitions of "clothed"), while some clubs in Canada offer naked lap dances. Usually, the best way to find out is to ask people who've frequented or worked in the clubs, or to visit them yourself.

Decide first which criteria are most important, based on your ideal fantasy and comfort limits: alcohol or no alcohol, full or partial nudity, lap dances, extras like peep booths—and then begin your search. Look in the back section of your local weekly paper or your nearest metropolitan weekly, or if you want anonymity, a publication from a city where you know no one at all. Make a list of your prospective clubs, and if you feel like doing research ahead of time, give them a call during daytime business hours. If a live person answers, ask if they have couples' specials. For first-timers, I recommend starting your strip club adventure with a higher-end club (which may bill itself as a "gentleman's club"). Most of these places are clamoring for heterosexual couples; they often let partnered women in free or give couples a two-for-one rate.

Expect to spend some money. Cover charges (just to get in the door) average around $10, but can climb as high as $40 on weekend nights—gentlemen's clubs can start at $40 on weeknights and go up from there. Don't try to barter with anyone, from doormen to dancers. Of course, you don't have to go to a fancy club on your first outing. You may enjoy adventure, want to hit several clubs, or have a recommendation from a friend. Either way, bring $50 to $200 in varying denominations (especially ones, fives, tens, and twenties) for your fun and games, and remember you don't have to spend it all to have a good time. You might just want to watch—and have rabid sex when you get home.

If you sit near the stage, the dancers will expect to be tipped, so have singles, fives, and tens ready—more if you're in an upscale club. If you don't plan to tip, give your seat up to the paying customers, and don't sit in any designated lap-dance seating unless you want a dance. When the women are done with their routines, they may circulate among the tables and ask if you want a lap dance. Always be polite, and if you see a girl you'd like to give you a lap dance, ask her.

In a very fancy club, you might spend hundreds of dollars, especially if you want to "try every ride at the carnival." Lap dances can range from $10 to $50 per song, and increase in price if performed in a private VIP area—which is sometimes just a curtained-off space with a chair. Find out ahead of time how much a lap dance costs, and whether a dancer charges double to lap-dance you both. If you decide to try a private show, agree on the price before you enter the room, and find out if you are required to purchase drinks. Using the private lap-dance areas comes with a minimum charge, such as $100 for three songs. Some clubs require or "suggest" that you purchase a bottle of champagne to drink in the booth, a suggestion that will cost you a ridiculous sum, from $20 to $200 a bottle. Sometimes the dancers ask you to buy them drinks, which is a scam many clubs employ to get you to buy overpriced drinks while the dancer just sits and sips non-alcoholic cocktails. Don't blow your money on overpriced booze—pay her to dance for you instead.

You may or may not have a fabulous time in strip clubs. The two of you could get turned on, spend some cash, get rubbed by naked girls (or boys), and barely make it out of the parking lot before you're dying to have sex. On the other hand, you might not like any of the women you see, find the atmosphere unnerving, or dislike the music, the bizarrely athletic pole dances, or the fake boobs, hair, and nails. Much like porn, your first strip-club experience might disappoint you, but remember that hundreds of alternative experiences—other clubs, dancers, atmospheres—await you.

Peep Booths

When you visit a peep booth, it's like having an exotic dancer give you an explicit masturbation show, to your specifications, but without a club atmosphere or any other distractions. Peep or "live girl" shows are just the ticket for couples who seek a focused, private interaction. Some strip clubs have peep booths, and you'll find "adult bookstores" that sell and rent porn and sex toys and offer peep booths in addition to private "arcade" booths where adult movies are shown. There are also establishments that feature only peep booths and "live girl" shows—while you may wonder what a "non-live girl" show might be, this designation means simply that it's a porn arcade.

Once in the peep booth, it's just the two of you—and a sexy woman behind the glass who wants to put on a show and help you get off. On your side of the glass there will be a stool or bench, a viewing window, and a slot for tips. To activate the show, you put money or tokens in the meter, and the glass will defog or the covering will slide up, revealing the sex worker for a specified period of time. The tip slot is where you'll pay the worker for the sex acts you'd like her to perform, and this is a separate transaction. Decide if she's your type immediately—often you'll see a picture of her before you go in, but have a code word or signal for each other that says, "not this one." Perhaps you might ask your partner if they "remembered to bring cash," and if the answer is no, then it's off to the next booth. You could also say, "Honey, I forgot my cash" as a way of signaling that you'd like to move on. Then excuse yourself politely.

When you come to the peep shows, be sure to bring as much as $100 in fives, tens, and a few twenties for a good show, and also bring any sex toys, lube, or safer-sex items you might want to play with. Of course, you don't need to plan on having sex in the booth, and you may not even like the experience or get turned on, but it's nice to have these items ready. It is a very good idea to bring a newspaper to sit or kneel on, in case the booth's previous occupants were erotic slobs. Insert your money, the girl will appear, and once you make eye contact, she will guide you through the activities you may request that she do for you; she might also suggest that you tip her.

Arcades Don't Have Video Games

Contrary to their names, adult bookstores don't really sell any books. Most sell adult novelties such as vibrators and wind-up hopping penises, sell and rent adult videos and DVDs—but make their daily bread and butter from their arcades. An arcade is a row (or multiple rows) of private movie booths with locking doors, where patrons can view porn, paid by the minute using tokens or cash. Also known as "jack shacks," this is where guys go to masturbate or give blow jobs to other guys, where prostitutes bring clients, and where adventurous couples come for quickies. While not an atmosphere for refined trysting, these seedy little booths often have what it takes to give a fantasy that gritty edge, and they make a great spot for an exceptionally nasty lunch-hour rendezvous.

Because it's illegal in most places to exchange money for sex acts, even where there is no direct sexual contact, you might have to play a bit of a guessing game until you and the performer settle on an agreeable amount for what you want her to do. She may be in a situation where she can be direct about sex acts and prices, or she may cryptically tell you that "you'll have a better party" if you're "more generous." Exchanges like this might sound like lines out of a bad porn movie or a cheesy crime novel, and they may lead to unintentionally hilarious "who's on first" conversations, but peep-booth workers need to be cautious to stay in business and do so by not overtly breaking any laws. Different peep operations will have different price structures. After your negotiations, all you have to do is pay, sit back, and enjoy your own personal, private sex show.

But *what* do you want her to do? Tell her what will turn the two of you on the most. In general, peep workers will strip and put on a terrific show of masturbating for you, a masturbation session that you can tailor to your fantasies. Sex toys, oral, vaginal, and sometimes anal play can all be on the menu, and she might even have vibrators, a paddle or whip, or other surprises in her bag of tricks. Peep workers are used to taking special requests, so if you want dirty talk, domination, submission, certain words or personas, fetishes such as smoking, or simply want to have her watch you, just ask. Get close to her—and to your partner—while you watch, and you can interact and talk dirty with her as she plays with herself. Play with each other, too, and take turns watching. You can give your lover a hand job, give your lover oral sex, mimic the woman behind the glass for a double show, and anything else that'll get you both off. If you liked the show, give the performer a nice tip.

Most peep shows feature women performers, but there are gay male peep shows, too. If you go to a gay club, make sure to ask beforehand if women are welcome as clients. You can expect to see a fat slice of hot and sweaty man-to-man action.

The biggest rules for all peep shows: Ignore other customers, and never, ever try to negotiate a better price.

Phone Sex

While phone sex is typically a one-on-one service, you and your partner both can play with the alluring voice on the other end of the line and have an incredible time together. Professional phone-sex workers are the masters of fantasy because all day long they listen to people's fantasies, tell fantasy stories, and do it all with the express purpose of getting the caller off. With a pro on the phone, one partner can talk while the other performs oral sex, or you can use a speakerphone to have sex while the phone sex operator talks dirty or directs the action. Also, you can conference on two separate cell phones, in two different locations, and masturbate with the phone-sex worker as your explicit instructor.

Phone sex is perfectly legal, though if calls are made at your workplace or not on your own phone you can get in trouble (read: fired), and keep in mind that it can get quite expensive. Look for services that advertise in the back of local weekly newspapers and reputable adult magazines. Phone-sex operations on the Internet are dicey, since literally anyone can put up a site in a few hours, so avoid websites unless you are referred by a satisfied customer. Make your decision based on the content of the ads, the prefix of the phone number, and the types of payment they accept—the more types they accept, the more established the service.

Number prefixes will dictate cost and content. Toll-free numbers start with 800, 866, 877, or 888, and will not appear on your phone bill. The charge goes to your credit card, though some services will allow third-party payments through online services or prepayment, where you send in a check or money order ahead of time. The FCC regulates 900 numbers and restricts what 900 operators may talk about. No credit card is required; the charge goes on your phone bill. International numbers start with 011 (except for Canada), and as with 900 numbers, no credit card is needed but the charge goes on your phone bill. International phone-sex calls can be very expensive, but if it's part of your specific fantasy or they offer a specialty you can't find domestically, it may well be worth it.

Paying by credit card is the norm, and the first person you talk to, either the dispatcher or sex operator, will ask for your credit card information before you get started. Make sure you ask their policy on sharing customer information and "opt out" if they do. Find out how the charge will appear on your credit card statement. If you don't want your charges to be seen by anyone who might get the bill, use a card whose bill will be seen by your eyes only. Even if the name of the service is innocuous, with minimal detective work anyone curious and smart enough can find out that you visited a phone-sex service.

When you call, be ready to tell the dispatcher or operator that you are a couple, exactly what you want, and how you plan to engage the phone-sex worker together—by speakerphone, multiple phones, or one on one. You'll need to be very specific, so writing details down in advance might help. Dispatchers route calls to workers who specialize in what you want, so telling them your specific fantasy will get you connected to the right person.

The operator will begin the call by asking you a few questions to determine your likes and to help you relax. During the call, don't be afraid to guide the operator by providing details and giving direction, and be participatory—even if it's by moans and grunts, the operator will need to know that he or she is on the right track. Tell them to talk dirtier, describe something in more detail, be more submissive or more cruel, or anything else you need more of. If the call is falling short of your expectations or your energy doesn't "click" with the operator, try changing fantasies to fit the mood or tone of your conversation, or end the call. You can also gently let the operator know that it isn't working for you and ask to be connected to someone else. You're paying by the minute for your fun and games, and the operator is on the clock, so make sure you're getting exactly what you want—and that both you and your partner get off.

Call Girls and Prostitutes

Perhaps you have a decadent fantasy of enacting a threesome with a high-priced call girl in a hotel suite in the middle of the afternoon—or your idea of calling for some "room service" is a full-service delivery for two. Or maybe you want to watch your lover having sex with a stranger in the backseat of your car. Want to give him or her a birthday present they'll never forget by turning that lesbian fantasy into reality? Trying out a threesome, voyeurism, same-sex contact, and other fantasies are all available for exploration with a hired pro. All of these fantasies are a phone call away, though you'll want to study up before you take the plunge into this exciting and sometimes perplexing territory.

Before you engage in actual sex with any new partner—as opposed to the minimal contact of strip clubs, peep booths, and phone sex—you'll need to take stock of your relationship and your expectations. Discuss what each of you wants and doesn't want to do or see. Read about jealousy in Chapter 5, "Threesomes, Foursomes, and Moresomes" to understand what emotions might come up, as well as how to deal with any unexpected feelings. This section will also give you tips for how to keep control of any multiple-partner situation at all times, and suggestions for code words that might come in handy in case either of you wants to stop or switch activities.

First and foremost, when engaging in sex with someone new, always use safer sex—see the chart in Chapter 12 for guidelines. Professional sex workers always use condoms—if they don't or won't, stop everything, pay them for their time, and find someone else.

Know the laws regarding prostitution in your city. Although prostitution is legal (and regulated) in many countries worldwide, in the U.S. it is legal in only a few counties. None of what I'm presenting here constitutes legal advice or condones the breaking of any laws. If you have legal concerns, talk to an attorney. But I can tell you how to have a good, safe encounter with a sex worker— in a locale or situation where it is legal.

You can choose from unlimited flavors of sex workers for your adventures. Before you go shopping you'll likely have a fantasy in mind that will dictate the type of pro you're looking for. For instance, you might want a quick and dirty encounter with a male or female street worker, in which case grittiness and coarseness will fit into your fantasy picture. Or you may see your ideal encounter taking place in a hotel room with a sex worker who fits a specific fantasy of sex with a stripper, a hustler, the girl-or-boy-next-door, or a cultivated courtesan.

Reputable online services such as www.Erosguide.com are national directories with phone-book-style entries featuring a wide variety of sex workers and verified photographs. Local weekly newspapers will have a plethora of ads in their back pages for escort services and individual. If an ad says "incall," you go to the sex worker's place; if the ad says "outcall," he or she comes to you, usually at a hotel room. Avoid any ads whose titles or wording suggests disrespect toward the sex workers themselves. Look for larger ads that are more costly to run and include terms like "upscale" and "elegant."

Make a list of possible agencies or individuals, and begin the process of elimination. For research purposes, call each prospect during daytime hours to see if they have a professional-sounding outgoing message, or are staffed during the day—two good signs. If the phone rings and rings, is answered by someone not associated with the escort service, or the number is not in service, cross it off your list. If you find one you might like, don't leave a message when you call—call back during evening business hours, usually from 8 P.M. to midnight.

When you are ready to make a "date," call the same day to set up your appointment, and have your hotel room already rented. If a woman is making the phone call, she should ask if the service entertains couples— this will eliminate confusion as to whether you're looking for a job and will let you know immediately if you've found a suitable agency. Say you'd like to make a couple's date; describe how you want the sex worker to look, whether you want a half hour, an hour, or longer (some will have a one-hour minimum), and be prepared to give your name, hotel, and room number.

If your scenario involves role play or costumes, be sure you let the sex worker know ahead of time that you'd like to pretend you're a schoolgirl, your lover likes to be told what to do, or that the two of you like to play doctor/nurse games, and so on—but don't discuss sex at this point. Mention any special requests, such as heavy makeup or no panties, and let the sex worker know if you have any items you'd like him or her to wear for you. Once your appointment is set, make sure you have safer-sex gear and any sex toys, lubricants, outfits, champagne, or other accoutrements that'll make your fantasy complete.

Some escorts will accompany you to a strip club (at their same hourly rate, of course), so the sky's the limit when it comes to combining your fantasies. Don't expect them to drink alcohol or do drugs with you—while some might, many are on the clock and have a full night of work ahead. And needless to say, never take anything with you that could make the situation worse if you encounter an undercover officer.

Do not expect the escort to engage in any S/M activities with you, though some independent escorts might be open to sessions that include professional dominance or submission. Information on pro dommes (and doms) can be found in Chapter 10, "Erotic Dominance and Submission: S/M Fantasies."

When your escort arrives, she or he may place a call to the agency to let them know they arrived safely, and may place or receive calls during or following the session for safety purposes. All parties will be very cautious in the beginning stages of the encounter; the sex worker will want to make sure you are not a cop, and you'll want to know the same. Since police officers generally can't take off their clothes, disrobing can be a good way to dispel everyone's fears. In all cases, the escort is never permitted to say that he or she will have sex for money, and you should never say that you will pay for sex acts of any kind. While this sounds like a convoluted way to negotiate your session, know that you can be more specific once clothes have come off and money (often called a "tip" or "donation") has been exchanged.

Learn your local laws regarding sex and prostitution, especially if you want to pick up someone off the street for your encounter. Having a hotel room ready is a good idea, since many streetwalkers won't have sex in your car because it's a good way to get arrested. You and your partner will want to cruise together in your car to find the streetwalker you like—he or she will be walking in a known prostitution area, and when you slow down, will come over to your car and ask if you want to "party." Don't discuss money until you get to the room. Trust your intuition—if it feels wrong, end it wherever you are.

In general, you can expect to pay an escort from $200 an hour upward, though rates for street prostitutes can start around $20–$50 for oral sex and $50–100 for intercourse, with street hourly rates averaging $60 to $200. Higher-class, independent escorts have rates for one and a half hours, two hours, dinner dates, overnights, and travel. Don't try to negotiate prices. Be polite, be on time, practice good hygiene, and bring cash. Always expect to use safer-sex practices. Respect the escort's limits, and if she is not to your liking, or isn't as described, thank her for her time, give her the required "tip," and send her on her way.

8

Public Sex

Public sex happens when you just can't wait, when your sex is a secret, when you can't get enough of each other and it "just happens"—or when the danger and excitement of being seen, watched, or caught in the act turns you on like a light switch. For some, the attraction to public sex comes from vivid memories and a desire to revisit an exciting, urgent, and focused sexual experience.

You may have seen movies depicting deliciously taboo sex in public places or read about it in erotica collections. You even may have had sex in a bar or movie theater, hands busy under or a cocktail table or hidden by a coat tossed over a lap. Many people are turned on by the idea of public sex. They find that clandestine sex in a public setting makes them feel like horny teenagers, and the possibility of being discovered only increases their arousal. Others are titillated by the prospect of simply being observed having sex.

This is sex on the sly, in situations involving varying degrees of tangible risk and the thrill that comes with it.

What's on the Menu

Public encounters are best suited for oral sex, because one partner can be the lookout while the other gets busy, oral sex can be performed relatively quickly, and a minimum of clothing is shed. Mutual masturbation is a discreet and delightfully dirty way to have public sex, with no need to remove clothes and simultaneous pleasure for both of you. Vaginal intercourse is next on the list of good choices for public spaces, because skirts and trousers fit together discreetly, hiding the real action. It's possible to appear as though you are merely standing very close when in fact you are engaging in penetration. Anal sex is last on the list, because it requires lots of extra lubrication, may not be a quick process, and if you are both wearing pants it will be pretty obvious to anyone who discovers you.

If possible, wear clothing that facilitates your sex act *du jour*. Skip the underwear altogether—or men can wear boxers with a wide-open fly and women can wear crotchless panties, or crotchless (or ripped open—yum!) tights or pantyhose under a skirt or dress. Go without a bra and wear a button-down shirt if you want to offer easy access to your breasts. Bring any safer-sex gear such as condoms, gloves, and dental dams, accessories such as lube and finger vibrators, and "pack" your strap-on under your clothing so that you are ready when the time comes. Condoms, dental dams, gloves, and lube all can be purchased in small, flat, discreet foil packets that slip easily into a shirt pocket—see the Resources chapter for ordering, and look for Slicks, a dental dam that comes in a single sterile foil packet.

Make absolutely sure that no one will see you. Yes, the threat of discovery is part of the thrill, but if someone sees you, you are involving that person in a sex act without his or her consent. This is not a good thing, not only because you could be apprehended by the police but because you might offend others or—even worse—unintentionally expose yourself to kids. Scope out your location before you actually do the deed. Pay a visit (or several) around the time of day or night you think you might have your adventure, and look around. If it seems possible that a passerby might chance upon the two of you locked in a sweaty tango, choose a different time or location. Think ahead about places to duck for cover, ways to camouflage your activity, or a story to tell an authority figure. But once you have taken these precautions, make your encounter as hot and fun as you can—public sex is a thrilling experience that can't be duplicated. Don't hold back!

Where to Do It

Seek out reliably secluded spots, such as a remote "parking" spot, a deserted natural area like a beach or forest, a vacant warehouse, or an empty movie theater. The days of joining the "mile high club" on airplanes are over—don't even consider it, because the consequences are now severe. Look around first, before you're horny:

- The backseat of a car (can be parked in any secluded spot).

- A quiet alley
- Public bathrooms (lock the door and choose a low-traffic time)
- Your backyard
- A public park at night
- An abandoned warehouse or waterfront
- A parking garage
- An empty movie theater
- Peep show booths
- A rooftop
- A boat
- A hotel balcony late at night
- A drive-in theater
- A stairwell
- Your workplace after hours—but have keys and a damn good excuse (and risk expulsion or even being fired)

Some alleys and parks in large cities are notorious as public sex spots. Use these places only if you are a local and are familiar with the area. If you must cruise, proceed with streetwise caution.

Role-Playing in Public

Sexual role-playing in public offers a multitude of delicious possibilities. In fact, you don't even have to engage in sex to add a charge to your role play if you wear a costume or enact your roles in public. Taking your roles into the big world outside the bedroom lends realism to your scene. You can speak to each other in character while sitting in a café, in a club, while walking down the street, or in the car on the way home. You might only be flirting, as a prelude to a scene waiting for you at home.

Or you might intend your entire scene to take place at a bar—and the alley behind it.

Wearing outfits in public that can pass as everyday clothing, such as uniforms or workwear, can be electrifying when only the two of you know that you're dressed that way for sex. Everybody else simply takes you at face value. This works well with typical adult roles such as construction worker, secretary, corporate executive, teacher, biker, repairman, deliveryman, sleazy photographer, or "stranger." You can make delivery calls, "cruise" your lover, go on a field trip, or drive off to your sexual rendezvous.

While it's possible in San Francisco to leave the house dressed as an adult schoolgirl and have no one bat a false eyelash—even if you're male—you'll want to exercise caution with certain roles in cities less accustomed to sexual variety. Doctors and nurses are sexy, but you don't want to have someone ask you for needed medical help. Police officers and firefighters don't take kindly to impersonators, and it goes without saying that pimps, human dogs, and adult babies shouldn't go out in public. You might be able to play a call girl or hooker at night, but err on the side of caution. Fake sex workers run all the same risks as real ones, and besides encountering police, hoodlums, and johns you might be confronted by real sex workers who don't want a new girl on their turf. Instead, find a hotel where you can discretely play the part of a callgirl, or pick up your "john" in a safe place, such as a restaurant.

Swinging

So many couples get turned on by the idea of being observed having sex that memberships in sex clubs and swingers' clubs are growing exponentially. While these clubs are predominantly venues where couples can swap partners and engage in multiple-partner sex, they also feature nonprivate rooms and thematic public spaces where members can observe and engage in all sorts of Bacchanalian sexual revelries. For anyone seeking a less risky public sexual encounter, sex clubs are just the ticket.

Swinging or "lifestyle" parties provide the safest way to try out public sex and multiple-partner fantasies. At these parties, you and your lover can have a sexual encounter while others watch, and you can be the voyeur for others engaging in a variety of sexual activities including orgies and the use of "love swings." Unlike a blow job in an alleyway or a quickie in a stairwell, swing parties give you an opportunity to flaunt your hot shared sex life to one or many appreciative voyeurs, at little risk—and you don't need to hurry or worry about being caught.

The world of swinging is vast, and it's growing every year. According to the North American Swing Club Association (NASCA), weekend events can pack in as many as 4,000 attendees. Open to heterosexual couples and single females, swinging is like a candy store for big kids who want to try a wide variety of sexual activities in environments that range from orgiastic house parties to "adult Disneyland" retreats with elaborate theme rooms. While in small suburban swing clubs you still might find 1970s-era throwbacks with mustaches and gold chains, most of the couples who make up the estimated ten million swingers in North America are in their 30s and 40s, are culturally hip and connected, have plenty of disposable income, and are quite comfortable with open and frank sexual displays.

Swinging, also called "the lifestyle," has been documented in America since the 1950s. The lifestyle finds expression in clubs geared toward couples. They welcome single women but generally discourage single men and are not at all open to male bisexuality—the rules vary from club to club. You can make a wide array of multipartner connections within the swinging community and its networks, for encounters that range from immediate sexual exchanges to ongoing relationships. You might find a few forms of light kink such as blindfolds at a swing party, but you'll seldom see alternative or S/M activities (or actual lesbian couples, for that matter)—this is an emphatically *vanilla* orgiastic crowd. You'll find websites for swinging clubs with schedules of parties and events, and magazines and newspapers catering to various swinging groups that consist largely of advertising space. National swinging organizations such as Lifestyles hold conventions, seminars, and classes on a range of sexual topics and organize swinging vacations, retreats, and cruises.

Swingers are typically middle-class folks who consider the openness and honesty of the lifestyle to be a healthy way of expressing sexuality. They hold certain traits and behaviors in high esteem, most notably respect, openness, tolerance, courtesy, and an outgoing personality—but the most important prerequisite is stability within an established relationship. Many find it refreshing to behave sexually in environments where there is an acceptance of different body shapes, ages, and sizes, and though male bisexuality is not considered part of swinging culture (or is forbidden outright), many women find this a safe, comforting, and relaxing milieu for exploring their bisexual urges.

Swing Parties

Swing events can be held as "on premises" parties, where sex happens at the gathering—usually a rented hotel, private mansion, rented resort, or cruise ship—or "off premises," where couples retreat to a hotel room or other locations away from the event for sex. In the U.S., most types of on premises parties are considered illegal, though some are legal in some states.

Most swing clubs carefully screen prospective couples and require an orientation session before new couples may attend their first party. The screening process can be as simple as a telephone conversation and a reservation/orientation requirement, or can be as intense as at one Bay Area club that requires an email describing yourselves and your interests, photos of the two of you, a phone conversation, and *then* a reservation/ orientation. Screening ensures that the hosts get a crowd that gels well, that partygoers will be respectful of each other and serious about the rules, and generally that single men are barred. At the orientation session, you'll be given a tour and briefed on the rules and etiquette of the party. On premises clubs that allow single men may admit them at higher fees and with a firm reservation requirement. Such events usually turn into parties where the men outnumber the women, but they can be a good place to fulfill "gang bang" fantasies with genuine strangers, in safety.

On premises swing parties held in private homes have a relaxed atmosphere and are hosted graciously by the homeowners. At these parties you'll find refreshments and spaces to meet and have sex with other couples, and the settings can range from spartan to decadent. The hosts may offer wine from their private cellars, lavish feasts, sex rooms bedecked with satin and gloss, a hot tub, porn viewing rooms, outdoor fire pits, and more—or the setting can be someone's suburban house with sheets on the windows and mattresses in every room. Off premises parties are usually held in dance clubs or bars that are closed to the public for the evening. Guests must apply for entrance and are interviewed prior to admission. These parties, held regularly in many areas, may have a theme to help break the ice, such as "naughty schoolgirl night." Off premises parties do not involve sexual participation (though the flirting can get explicit); rather, they serve as places where couples can hook up to meet for sex away from the club.

Swinging Etiquette

Making reservations is the typical protocol for attending swing events, and it is proper to cancel your reservation if you can't make it. Etiquette and rules vary (your orientation will give you the real lowdown). The following are some general rules that should never be broken—breaking the rules at swing parties will get you blacklisted.

Rule number one is never to discuss your experiences or involvement in the clubs with anyone outside the lifestyle, and never "out" anyone you see at the parties. Second, there is no pressure on anyone to participate, ever—do not press, and expect that no will always mean no. Three, all couples arrive as a couple, participate as a couple, and leave as a couple. Four, don't do or bring drugs. Some smaller private (noncommercial) parties may look the other way at pot smoking. And five, it is generally considered rude to drink to excess, have arguments in public spaces, or talk while people are having sex.

As a social activity centered on parties and events, swinging relies on people getting to know each other, and it's a natural outlet for the flirtatious and the chatty. Generally, you'll socialize with a couple, flirt a little, discuss each other's swing styles, and then you get to play. "Closed swinging" means that one partner chooses not to be around while their lover is having sex with others; "open swinging" means they both participate; and "soft swinging" denotes heavy petting with others but no sex. Many clubs have a rule that prohibits voyeurs from asking to join couples already engaged in sex, meaning that onlookers can participate only if expressly invited. Typically the cost to attend is around $80 per couple (with two women also considered a couple) and $20 for a single woman.

You don't have to have sex if you go to a swing party; it's perfectly okay to simply watch, or just flirt. For your first party or event, plan on going solely as an observer—many other newcomers will be doing the same. Just watching your first time out is a great way to see if swinging is for you and to see how couples and singles interact.

What if one member of a couple is more attracted than the other to someone at the party? The conversation—and flirtation—that results from that situation is fascinating. For instance, the man in couple "A" might find the woman in couple "B" attractive. He flirts with her, and they find they share a mutual sexual interest. So Mr. A indicates his interest to his partner, Ms. A, who may fancy Ms. B—she may desire her for a threesome, or she may want to watch Ms. B having sex with her man. Perhaps she thinks Ms. B's partner, Mr. B, is quite alluring. That's when things get really interesting.

Mr. and Ms. A flirt with Ms. B, who then asks Mr. B if he fancies the A's. If everyone is enjoying the flirtation, the two couples continue chatting and flirting, and as the chemistry begins to simmer, the talk turns to the matter of a possible sexual encounter. If this sounds clinical or awkward, try it in a dimly–lit bar, over drinks with a gorgeous couple or on a crowded dance floor, or while watching others do the same. In the right context, the exchange may prove to be a powerful aphrodisiac.

Finding the club that's right for you might take a bit of research. Swing and sex clubs don't advertise, and sometimes the club you're looking for seemingly pops up out of nowhere. Joining an organization such as NASCA can get you connected to a network of clubs, events, magazines, and a variety of resources from seminars to conventions—membership in NASCA costs $50 per couple for one year. When you find a few clubs that sound intriguing, give them a call (look in the Resources chapter for ways to find clubs in your area). Find out their hours of operation, and ask how big a crowd they get. While bigger isn't necessarily better, variety is the spice of this particular lifestyle—initially, try to visit clubs with more than two dozen attendees. Or, if you enjoy male bisexuality, crave sexual diversity, like a little kink with your club, or want to see how the rest of the sexual underground plays, try out sex parties outside "the lifestyle."

Alternative Sex Parties

Through a friend of a friend, I managed to get myself on an email list run by a loosely organized group of people who were regulars at the same dance club and had decided to organize their own sex parties. I watched the email postings in fascination, but never attended. From that list, I was put on another list for a very different kind of sex party, where the attendees were devotees of fantasy and fetish, liked storybook themes, and dressed up in ways that make those Halloween stripper-schoolgirl outfits look like Cinderella's daytime tatters. I was way too intrigued to protest being put on this list.

Finally, I decided to go to one of these parties. After spending a few hours at San Francisco's famous S/M event, the Folsom Street Fair, my date and I wandered to an innocuous looking door on a side street, only to have it swing open and find ourselves greeted by a tipsy drag queen, bedecked in a rubber corset dress. We were asked for a password, then sent upstairs and asked for our email confirmation information. We paid the nominal $15 entry fee, checked our coats, and watched as one girl received a spanking before she even handed her coat to the attendant!

Wandering the huge Victorian, we saw that the rooms had been converted into open spaces including a dance floor, theme rooms decorated with pillows and stuffed animals, a lounge, two bars, an S/M playspace with dungeon equipment, and a theater where performances were ongoing through the evening. A table offered drinks, dishes of peanuts, and bowls of sanitary towelettes hilariously packaged with instructions on use as "facial come wipes."

People smiled and greeted us—and the crowd wasn't your Uncle Fred's swing couples, no ma'am. These people, dressed to the nines in corsets, rubber, leather, sexy fairy outfits, priest costumes, and more, were a mostly boy–girl coupled crowd, but with butch dykes, femme lesbians, tranny boys and tranny girls, and an assortment of gay men, they defied stereotypes. Everyone socialized, danced, sipped, and snacked. As the evening progressed, the S/M playspace filled with people, and the pillow-lined rooms heated up as couples took their flirtation to the next level. It was a subtle, gradual change. At one point my date and I went to the dance floor and passed an empty room; on our way back, we saw a beautiful blonde in a pink rubber tutu being serviced—and servicing—two men in uniforms, all of them laughing and flirting, while a same-sex couple on pillows watched the trio and took turns performing oral sex on each other. In the S/M space, couples, triples, and larger groups were kissing, tying each other up, spanking, and teasing—and having sex.

Non-swinging sex parties encompass a wider range of sexual expression than swing clubs limited to primarily heterosexual, vanilla sex. Some underground affairs, like the one described above, can take a bit of work to find, but are well worth the effort if public sex in an alternative atmosphere is what you're seeking. Look for public events that cater to bisexual, pansexual, and fetish audiences. Pay a visit to www.sexuality.org for a primer on throwing your own sex party, a popular option among sex-positive pansexuals. The underground route isn't the only one available—most major cities have parties and clubs open to the public that cater to kinky couples and singles; they are not difficult to find. Read all about it in Chapter 10, "Erotic Dominance and Submission: S/M Fantasies."

The View from Paris

BY ALISON TYLER

The view from the balcony overlooking Paris's residential 13th *arondissement* took in romantic rooftops, a breathtaking candy-pink sunset, and a lone young man in a firecracker-red T-shirt watching the two of us with unwavering interest. Josh saw him first. "Look down, Carla," he said, his hand under the strap of my gauzy silver nightgown. "Over there..."

I looked in the direction he was indicating, and that's exactly the moment when Josh slid the straps over my bare arms and pulled my forties-style movie-star nightgown past my naked breasts to the curve of my hips.

"Josh..." I said, crossing my arms over my full breasts. "He's watching."

"That's what I was telling you," my new husband said, nuzzling the back of my neck as his hands removed mine from my breasts. His fingers took over, teasing my nipples as he continued to kiss along the nape of my neck. "He's been there every evening."

And so had we. This was our new tradition, to slip into night clothes in the late afternoon, waking just when the sun went down to catch a sunset romp out on the balcony. We'd felt exposed, yet oddly protected, being up on the fifth floor of the apartment we'd rented for our honeymoon. Now I knew that we weren't protected at all. Josh seemed thrilled by this prospect, and as his fingers relentlessly played over my breasts, I relaxed into the idea, as well. We were in Paris, after all. Nobody knew us. None of our normal, everyday activities were in play here. Our entire routine was topsy-turvy in the most pleasurable way. We no longer started our morning with a healthy meal of oatmeal and OJ. In Paris, we had croissants at 10, then lingered over filling lunches around 1, not bothering to even think about dinner until 9 in the evening. At the time of day when we'd usually be facing rush hour traffic, we made love.

Now Josh moved to my side and turned me so that I was facing him. We were still easily visible to our naughty neighbor, and I kept that in mind as Josh began to kiss my breasts. He used one hand to palm my right tit while he suckled from the left. Then he switched activities, so no part of my body felt left out. As his mouth worked me over, I thought about the scene we'd admired the night before. Josh had suggested an evening at The Crazy Horse, and we'd enjoyed the erotic art of the women dancing and exposing themselves to us. Was I crazy enough on Paris's open attitudes to let myself be a woman on display? It seemed that I was.

When I didn't protest, or try to pull Josh back into the apartment, he slowly undid the tie at the back of my nightgown that held the dainty fabric in place at my hips. With one pull of the lace, the nightgown slid in a ripple of lovely silk to my ankles.

Here I was, a woman of satiny skin and curves, bathed in the pink glow of the heavens and admired by two sets of eyes: my husband and the man in the bright red shirt. And while I've always adored being on display for my man, it was the stranger's eyes that made me tremble.

Who was he? What did he think about my body? Was he turned on by my feminine curves or by Josh's hard and lean physique?

These thoughts and a multitude of others were still running through my mind when Josh bent me over the railing and began to kiss between my thighs from behind. I felt the slight breath of cool evening air surround me and the warmth of his tongue and lips against my pussy. The sensations were intensely arousing—being outside while behaving in the most intimate of ways has always been a turn-on for me, a fantasy I don't usually get to indulge in. Josh and I live in such a small town that the disgrace of being caught playing in public is too much to live down. Too much for us to ever get more frisky then a little petting in a parking lot every once in a while.

But we weren't in our small town anymore. We were in Paris, and I gazed into the room owned by a stranger and imagined I could see the yearning in his face, the desire in his eyes, the bulge in his slacks.

Josh made me thoroughly wet with his naughty kissing games, and then he stood and slid his pajama bottoms down, parted my thighs, and entered me. I closed my eyes for one moment, basking in the dreamy feeling of being taken by my husband. But I had to open them again quickly so that I could stare at our audience. I've read that when you're on stage, you're supposed to choose one person to focus on, to do your show for that single selected audience member. I'd chosen mine, and he seemed deeply honored, leaning into his windowsill, anxious to catch every act of our very personal show.

My handsome husband fucked me from behind for as long as he could take it, and then turned me around, lifting me into his embrace and bouncing me up and down on his glorious cock. I couldn't watch from this position, but I didn't mind. I could feel the stranger's eyes on my body, and my pussy responded by tightening and releasing rapidly, connecting with Josh, contracting on him.

When I came, it was as if there were three of us right there on the balcony: me and Josh and a man whose name I didn't know, but whose willing participation took me higher than I ever had been before. I cried out, not bothering to try to stifle the sounds of my pleasure, and Josh responded by coming right away, holding me tightly to his body as he filled me up. We stayed connected, my legs around his waist, until a shiver ran through me and Josh set me down on the tiny balcony once again.

As I reached for my discarded nightgown, I thought about our choices for honeymoon locations, and our decision to come to Paris, a place renowned for its sights. It turns out the most exciting view Paris had to offer was us.

Fetishes

When you hear the word *fetish*, I'll bet you have one of three reactions. You think of fetish fashion—shiny, skintight outfits made of rubber or leather, tight-laced corsets or shiny buckles, much like the suits worn by Edward Scissorhands and Catwoman. Maybe you imagine the fringes of sexuality cranked up to their highest levels—people humping balloons, crushing bugs with their high heels, riding elaborately costumed, sexualized human ponies. Or you blush excitedly, revisiting in your mind the one thing that turns you on the very most.

Apart from fetish community publications, little is written about fetishes that doesn't sensationalize them or psychoanalyze them as bizarre and deviant practices pursued by only a handful of people—despite the numerous conventions, well-attended events, magazines and newsgroups with hundreds of thousands of sub-scribers, and fetish fashion boutiques all over the world. Indeed, in many minds, people with fetishes occupy the freakish end of the gene pool when it comes to sex; they politely relegate fetishes to a hidden world where far-out sexual tastes can be satisfied. The truth is, when you look at cultural stereotypes of "normal" sex, pretty much anything you do outside of heterosexual, missionary-position intercourse can be considered "deviant," and in reality, everyone has a fetish of one kind or another—a sexual position, a particular eye or hair color, a body part. Nowhere in the world of sexual expression do humans become more playful—and their tastes more unpredictable—than in the world of fetish.

A sexual fetish is an object, manner of dress, or specific scenario that takes on a magical quality and a deeper meaning, and is absolutely required for satisfy-ing sexual release. The item or scenario becomes that person's most reliable sex toy, and as we all know when it comes to orgasm, if you find something that works, you mine it for all it's worth. Seldom is there a rational explanation for why an individual is attracted to a cer-tain pair of shoes, wearing restrictive and beautiful corsets, watching women smoke in the nude, or popping bal-loons during sex. We have many culturally accepted explanations as to why big boobs and huge cocks are fashionable sexual fetishes, but people with fetishes out-side the norm get stigmatized. This is tough to cope with when you or your lover has a fetish you'd like to share.

Fetishes do not discriminate based on gender, race, or class. Fetishes are not good or bad, male-only or female-only. Many female fetishists eroticize the same objects in the same manner as men, though we tend to see more of the male perspective on the Web and in magazines because men are considered the primary consumers of pornography. No one gets hit on the head, as in the movies, and wakes up with a fetish. Clinical explanations about fetishes evolving from childhood experiences and Freudian experiences with parental nudity reek of the same contrived stink as theories about homosexuality from the 1950s. As articulate as fetishists typically can be regarding their obsessions, sometimes there simply is no rational explanation for a given fetish.

Fetish fashion and its connoisseurs make a couture designer's obsessions seem trite. Leather, shiny rubber, PVC, plastics, liquid latex, corsets, stilettos and fantastically high heels, stockings, and more occupy this highly sexualized realm of style. Fetish fashion is a huge industry, especially in North America and Europe. The sexuality underlying "fetish" blends well with S/M practices and Gothic style—and it's common to see fetish events that are also S/M play parties. For the moneyed rubberist, corset-wearer, or hard-core human animal fetishist, the fashion has become a fetish unto itself: The women at San Francisco's corset house Dark Garden have told me tales of fetishists with custom-made rubber suits for every imaginable occasion, including a rubber undertaker's suit. Formal fetish balls and conventions are typically high-fashion events with strict dress codes that embrace a wide variety of fetishes—as long as the revelers dress in full fetish gear.

A Fetishist Looks Just Like You

People with fetishes are generally articulate, well-read, and computer savvy, with theories about their fetishes and a very serious sense of self-control about the way they conduct their sex lives. Many feel they cannot share their fetish with their loved ones, and discreetly set aside a time and place where they can find fulfilling release with their fetish, avoiding the risk of offending people they care about. Most fetishists who visit professional fantasy-makers such as dominatrixes have a healthy understanding of negotiation and boundaries. While many fetishists have healthy, happy sex lives with their lovers, others must partition off their sexual fetishes from their relationships. This can be isolating.

We live in a culture that sees masturbation—a healthy, normal sexual practice—as shameful and degrading, so it's no surprise that people with fetishes are reluctant to share them, even with their lovers. Single fetishists can attempt to network over the Internet, finding others who share their tastes, but, like a night out at a single's bar, it can be a routine of disappointment. So they are compelled to gamble, dating people they find attractive but dreading the moment of revelation when their new partner may reject them upon discovering the fetish. Opening up in a relationship and sharing your inner-most sexual workings with a partner you don't want to lose can be so frightening that many don't risk it. Telling anyone about a fetish presents the risks of rejection, shame, loss, and heartbreak.

Fetishes, by and large, are harmless—within the commonsense limits that apply to any act of pleasure, of course. But a fetish can become harmful when keeping it a secret begins to isolate one partner in a relationship. Fetishes come from the id, that bountiful and capricious source of sexual energy, and because they seldom have an explanation (fetishes are not chosen), they also can-not be "cured" or made to just "go away." In a relation-ship, a fetish can cause problems when the fetishist feels bad about keeping it a secret; when the fetish interferes with other parts of the fetishist's life; and when the fetishist's partner finds the fetish disturbing or distasteful—or worse, sees the fetish as competition. Some people with fetishes can't reach orgasm unless their fetish is involved, and this may make a lover feel inadequate.

If you or your lover has a fetish and is having a difficult time understanding how to work the fetish into your shared sex life, read this chapter together and discuss it. Also read "When Fantasies Make You Feel Bad," in Chapter 1, and "Talking to Your Partner" and "When Your Partner Is Reluctant," both in Chapter 3. Be sure to let your lover know that your fetish is the only surprise you've got up your sleeve—and take care to pay equal attention to the sex you share with your lover as you do to your fetish, and when you do bring your fetish into your shared encounters, don't let your lover feel left out. Reassure your partner that you are more aroused by them than by your fetish—this will be their number one concern.

Finding out that your partner has a fetish might be upsetting at first. It's easy to wonder if your lover has been keeping sexual secrets all along. But remember that your lover is entrusting you with their scariest—and most sexually exciting—secret. Understand that his or her arousal from a certain scenario or object is in no way a substitute for you—on the contrary, your lover is saying that adding you to the fetish dynamic will make them feel sexually complete (and make for some very hot sex that you both can enjoy). Don't see the fetish as a rival, or something you have to compete with for your partner's love and affection; instead, use the fetish as a tool to enhance and intensify their sexual arousal with you. A fetish shared by two, after all, is a very specialized sex toy, one you cannot buy at any sex boutique.

How to Have Sex with a Fetishist

Most folks probably don't know they have a fetish for certain objects, devices, or scenarios, but those who do make it easy to get the most out of the steamy sexual encounters you can have with a fetish. Of course, due to the very specific nature of sexual fetishes, the nuances of sex involving fetishes will be tailored to each fetish. Classic types of fetishes are discussed later in this chapter. To get you started, here are some guidelines for having hot fetish sex:

For the Fetishist

- Explain exactly what turns you on about your fetish so your lover can utilize the information to the utmost.
- Split your attention between your fetish and your lover. Err on the side of giving your partner more attention than the fetish. Do not behave selfishly.
- Do everything you can to keep your lover from feeling threatened by your fetish.
- Give your partner sexual pleasure in return for honoring your fetish. Get your partner off in whatever way they like best.
- Be a good lover. Your fetish is just another sex toy for you both to share.
- Be supportive. Tell your lover how hot they look, how aroused they make you feel, and afterward, all the things they did that made you see stars.
- Remember that you're not alone. Your lover wants to be there for you. And there are support groups and message boards on the Internet for even the most obscure fetish.

For the Partner of the Fetishist

- Find out in as much detail as possible what turns your lover on about the fetish item, scenario, or behavior. Ask questions: Do you rub the shoe all over their body or wear it? Do you want to eat from it or crush things with it?
- Have the fetishist show you what he or she likes to do when they masturbate.
- Let your lover know whether or not their fetish turns you on. If it doesn't, be prepared to say how you would prefer that they bring you to orgasm. Don't let sexual attention go unreciprocated, or you will feel resentful.
- If you're in a relationship, actively explore elements of your partner's fetish that excite or arouse you. You may discover that you enjoy having power and control over your partner's orgasm, so much that you *do* get turned on by sitting in cheesecake or posing with a cigarette. Or you may just enjoy seeing your lover get so sexually worked up.
- Push it. Does your lover get hard at the sight of rubber panties? Tease them, taunt them, rub the panties in their face, make their arousal as excruciating as possible before you give them what they want. Work it!
- Fetishists who like having something rubbed on them can be forbidden to masturbate as you rub them with the object, and you can take your time masturbating them to orgasm.
- Know your limits and boundaries. If it's too strange for your present tastes, talk about it. Never do anything you're uncomfortable with or might feel bad about later.

- Some fetishes involve images, photographs, or videos. This is a great opportunity for hand jobs and fun sexual positions.
- Be open to new and unusual experiences, and be playful about sex. It's like being able to be a kid all over again, but as consenting adults who can think of sexy twists to playtime red hot.
- Remember that you're not alone—a great many people have a lover with a fetish. There may well be a million fetishists in the U.S., possibly thousands with your lover's particular fetish. You can seek out Web communities and message boards for support.

Classic Fetishes

If it exists, someone has eroticized it. The fetishes, gear, and scenarios listed below include some of the more popular and notorious fetishes. Apologies if I excluded your fetish—this list is simply a sample. Although the list categorizes fetishes into subject areas, they often overlap. You might find yourself with a shoe fetishist who likes crushing and wants you to smoke while you step on them in spiked heels—three fetishes in one. Fetishists spend a lot of masturbation time fantasizing about their fetishes, and while some of the ones listed below may sound outrageous or impossible, remember that the fetish is a fantasy: It is not expected to become reality. Fetish fantasies often involve a relationship with a certain object (the fetishist masturbates with the shoes), or the object's relationship with another person (you are the one wearing the shoes, teasing and tormenting your lover into erotic rapture).

For links to fetish websites, both commercial and personal, see Chapter 13, "Resources."

Amputees

Amputees and their devotees are people who fantasize about missing limbs or digits. The most common sexualization is masturbating while looking at pictures of amputees or amputee porn. It can also be a fetish for prosthetics. For interesting perspectives on these fetishes, see www.amputeeonline.com/amputee/acrotomophile.html.

Balloons

"Looners" like to get off in a number of ways. They might look at pictures of clothed women popping balloons, hump large balloons until they pop, or watch sexy people blow up balloons; or they might wish to be encased in a balloon. The gallery at www.loonerz.com is worth a look.

Bandages

Bandage fetishes and Japanese "broken doll" fetishes focus on medical casts, bandages, traction, braces, and other bandage-type wearables. In Japan, the broken doll is typically a schoolgirl "hit by a car" and depicted in a full-body cast wearing her schoolgirl uniform with skirt lifted and panties showing, or no panties at all. A bandage fetishist might like to wear bandages, have sex with a bandaged person, or look at pictures of bandaged people. See photograph collections like Nobuyoshi Araki's *Tokyo Lucky Hole* and Romain Slocombe's *City of Broken Dolls*.

Body Modification

When an individual becomes sexually excited by modifying their own body through piercing, cutting, branding, corset training, tattooing, or other methods, they have a body modification fetish. Alternatively, they may become aroused by performing body modification on others, or by looking at photographs. There are numerous books and websites devoted to body modification in all its permutations—for starters, have a look at *Body Play* magazine and the website of body modification practitioner and performance artist Fakir Musafar: www.bodyplay.com.

Body Parts

These are fetishes for a particular part of the anatomy, such as the neck, navel, breasts, anus, thighs, hands, or elbows. "Big breast" fetishists make up a significant population, and tend to eroticize anything bigger than a D-cup. There are many foot and leg fetishists (see "Feet/Legs," below). The fetishist might like to touch the special body part, gaze at it, or have it rubbed on them during masturbation.

Clowns

A clown fetish can be stranger than fiction. This category includes fetishists with an innately twisted sense of humor who like to dress as clowns, usually with an adult variation such as topless, with a strap-on, or partially clothed in lingerie. Ouchy the Clown is San Francisco's premier clown pro dom and male escort. No, really. Read Cara Bruce's article "Bedding Bozo" at www.eros-guide.com/articles/2002-10-23/beddingbozo/.

Corsets and Corset Training

The old-fashioned Victorian corset has seen some literally breathtaking updates in the past fifty years. The feeling of being laced up, the restriction of motion, and the hourglass shape the corset provides are powerful to a corset fetishist. Some may prefer to wear the corset, see them being worn, or undergo corset training, where a corset is worn for extended periods, permanently changing the shape of the waistline. See the Resources chapter for magazines, books, and websites about fetish fashion that include corsetry.

Crushing

Fetishizing the act of crushing or being crushed takes place largely in the imagination. High heels crushing bugs, hands, feet, and tiny people are all popular crushing fantasies. Individuals into crushing might like to watch, or they may pretend to be the hapless creature being crushed. In 1998, as a result of a case involving a man who created and sold videos depicting small animals being crushed (he was arrested on animal cruelty charges), the U.S. Congress banned interstate trafficking of crush videos. In 2002, Britain followed suit, sending four crush video makers (one male, three female) to jail.

Diapers/Infantilism

People who like to wear adult diapers can become both aroused and comforted by the experience, or enjoy feeling helpless (as a baby), or humiliated. Fetishists who are into infantilism become big babies, in effect, and might enjoy being diapered, breastfed, pampered, given toys and a playpen, spanked, or having their diapers changed. A complete resource for adult baby gear, from diapers to *Diaper Tales Magazine,* can be found at http://store.yahoo.com/dpf/ind.html (don't be fooled by the baby themes—this resource is exclusively for adults).

Enemas

Enema fetishists are after a bit more than that clean feeling, though they are probably in impressive colonic health. These people enjoy receiving or administering enemas (anal douches), as punishment, pleasure, or humiliation. They might want to play it as a medical scene. Enema kits can be purchased at drugstores, and should be administered near a toilet. Find medical fetish enema gear at www.medicaltoys.com.

Fantasy Creatures

Far-out space creatures, mythical beasts, and animals with special powers make these fetishists hot and rarin' to go. They might like to impersonate a fantasy creature and fight or have animal sex, or they may enjoy playing the helpless human, or having you play the helpless human. See Chapter 4, "Role Play," for suggestions.

Fat People

A number of individuals find fat people, their clothing, or eating habits arousing. Fat fetishists get turned on by very large people, usually women, and they often take measurements as part of foreplay. Some like to be "feeders," helping their lust objects increase in size. If you're not their fat ideal, don't try to become it—have fun with images and porn instead. Check out the wonderfully unapologetic book *Fat? So!*, by Marilyn Wann, and a website with sexy fat-positive links, www.fatso.com. Another great resource is the guidebook *Big Big Love: A Sourcebook on Sex for People of Size and Those Who Love Them,* by Hanne Blank.

Feet/Legs

A surprisingly common fetish is sexy feet or legs. The fetishist will have very personal ideas of perfection when it comes to the shape of the arch, the look of toenails, skin tone, etc. If you're not Mr. or Ms. ideal feet, treat yourself to pedicures and foot or leg pampering to spiff 'em up. Your fetishist may prefer to do that for you. They may get excited taking care of your feet—touching, rubbing, kissing, sucking, licking, or just looking at them. So many options! *Leg Show* (www.legshow.com) is a terrific print magazine dedicated to leg and foot fetishes, and routinely features well-known fetish photographers.

Furry Animal Costumes

"Furries" represent a population large enough to hold their own conventions. These merry "furverts" dress in the over-sized costumes one might see in an amusement park, though many of them have easily accessible genital openings. Some like to hump or have sex with others in these costumes, others only like to wear the costumes (no sex), and many playact as the actual animal charac-ters in a sexual context. One clever fellow I interviewed created his own dog costume with a snug, silicone-lined tube to fit his penis into. A very thorough furry lifestyle FAQ and link list can be found at PeterCat's Furry Info Page, www.tigerden.com/~infopage/furry, and even more links at Tigercat's Big Page of Furry Links: www.tigerden.com/Sites/furlinks.html.

Gender-Specific Clothing

Some people get hot looking at, wearing, masturbating with, or having others wear gender-specific clothing. This might include clothing typically worn by men, such as a necktie or boxer shorts, or typically worn by women, such as stockings, bra, garters, panties, dresses, skirts, and so on. Some people can become highly fix-ated on a particular item, so you both might wind up playing with a jockstrap, a sweaty white sports bra, or white cotton panties.

Giantesses

A fetish for big, tall women. Not just women over six feet, we're talking about the fifty-foot-tall woman. Sometimes these fetishists like to be overpowered or "crushed" underfoot, sat on, or trampled. This is a fun role-play and dirty talk opportunity, where the giantess can masturbate her fetishist while she squishes his tiny body between her breasts, puts him in her mouth, inserts him vaginally or anally, or crushes him with her spiked heel. Usually found in online directories under "macrophilia" and "giantesses." A gold mine of images and resources on giant women and tiny men can be found at Giantess Magic, Inc., www.gts2.net/.

Hair

People with a hair fetish become aroused by body hair such as pubic or armpit hair, or they eroticize head hair—long, short, cutting it, shaving it. Your lover might like to touch your hair, be smothered by it, look at pictures of it, or masturbate with it. People seeking porn with hairy woman and men might search for nudist magazines from the "classic" era (1960s and '70s). *Leg Show Magazine* often features women with copious pubic hair, as does *Hair to Stay* magazine (www.hairtostay.com), and you can find a large list of links at the woman-run www.hairywebsites.com.

Human Animals/Training

Ponies, dogs, cats, farm animals—there are thousands of fetishists worldwide who relish their lives as erotic animals. They are groomed, trained to perform, receive behavioral punishment, "bred" with other animals, and outfitted with costumes and gear to make them more like the animal they identify as.

Inflation

The fetishist gets off inflating body parts with saline and looking at photos or illustrations of fantastical (and often impossible) bodily inflation (usually involving a woman's breasts). Not for casual experimentation. Rubber inflation fetishists enjoy wearing rubber suits and having them inflated with air, or wearing inflatable masks that obstruct the senses.

Machines

People who become aroused by machinery, by using machines as sex toys, or who secretly identify as machines have a machine fetish. They may become a machine, or become aroused when a partner is revealed to be a machine (humanized machines may fall under the "human doll" category). This is an imagery-driven fetish, but sex machines that vibrate and penetrate (such as the expensive Sybian) can be purchased online. See www.fuckingmachines.com and www.sybian.com.

Mannequins/Human Dolls

Similar to the human machine fetish, this is a fetish for inanimate humanoids, played either by you or by your lover. Mannequins and human dolls can be dressed and undressed, positioned, admired, and used sexually without protest.

Medical

Medical fetishes are another common fascination. Doctor and nurse uniforms, medical procedures (especially sexual ones), medical equipment, and anything else related to the hospital or doctor's office apply here. Yes, even dentistry. For scene ideas, see Chapter 4, "Role Play" and Chapter 10, "Erotic Dominance and

Submission: S/M Fantasies." Get your medical fetish gear at www.medicaltoys.com.

Midgets

A fetish for midgets, dwarves, and smaller-than-average people. May include watching porn, looking at pictures, role-playing midget sex, or having different types of sexual encounters with midgets.

Panties

More than just a gender-specific item of clothing, panties exert a special power for many people, making this fetish one of the most common. Looking up skirts, getting glimpses, touching, smelling, being smothered, having panties stuffed in the mouth like a gag, stealing panties, and masturbating with them can all be exciting for panty fetishists. You'll find plenty of panty porn in *Leg Show Magazine* and in explicit erotic photo books by photographer Roy Stuart.

Pregnancy/Lactation

This fetish includes becoming aroused by pregnant women, by the sight of breastfeeding, being breastfed, and fantasies about nursing from giant breasts. It may be a part of infantilism fantasies, but generally involves masturbating and looking at pictures or videos. You can pretend to nurse your partner easily enough while they masturbate, or you masturbate them or employ creative sexual positions for penetration.

Rubber

Rubber fetishists are a refined breed. These people eroticize the smell, feel, and look of rubber garments, which can include rubber isolation suits and masks. The fetishist either wears the rubber or dresses their lover in it, and it might be sexualized in dozens of creative ways, including bondage, inflation (filling with air), and isolation, where the senses are restricted by masks, breathing is conducted through tubes, and the whole body is encased in layers of specially made tight rubber garments and mummy bags. Some find merely wearing or seeing a rubber dress, corset, or tight-fitting shiny garment to be arousing.

Scars

This refers to arousal by scars or scar tissue, such as old wounds, surgery scars, or vaccination scars. Scar fetishists might like to look at, touch, hear you talk about, masturbate on, or rub themselves on the scar. You can visit a theater makeup store and make a titillating road map on your body of elaborate scars for your fetishist to find, and change them for each encounter. David Cronenberg's film *Crash* features a scar fetish theme throughout.

Shoes

Shoe fetishists are another very common breed. Sarah Jessica Parker and her thousands of Manolo Blahniks aside, shoe fetishists typically fetishize a specific type of shoe. They may collect them to look at or masturbate with, get aroused when another person wears them, ask you to do something with the shoes while they masturbate (such as put a shoe in their mouth or step on them with the shoes), prefer having your regular style of sex while one of you is shoe-clad, or simply get turned on when you wear a certain pair of your own shoes.

Sleeping

I know you're wondering: How can someone have a fetish if they're asleep? Silly, a sleep fetish is where the fetishist gets turned on by being sexually used while they're asleep, becomes aroused by watching others sleep (clothed or not), or entertains fantasies about having sex with someone who is asleep. This is an easy and fun one to play with—good luck trying to stay "asleep" when you're turned on. A nexus of sleep fetishism can be found at www.sleepyrealm.com.

Smoking

The act of smoking, especially when performed by someone the fetishist finds sexually attractive, is a powerful aphrodisiac for the smoking fetishist. For them, nude smokers, novice smokers, and the acts of lighting up, puffing, blowing smoke, ashing, and extinguishing can be a huge turn-on. This may require a small chain-smoking session when you have sex, but if you don't smoke, it's easy to fake by drawing the smoke into your mouth and slowly releasing it with air from your lungs. High-class porn director Andrew Blake often includes smoking in his many long and languid, fetish-tinged girl–girl sex scenes. Check out the smoking fetish magazine *Smoke Signals* at www.smokesigs.com.

Stuffed Animals

Covered in fake fur and stuffed with—stuffing, stuffed animals conjure up images of childhood animal-companion fantasies, and are many people's first masturbation toys. People who like stuffed animals ("Plushies") may be revisiting these feelings, but they also may enjoy the feeling of the toys on their body or genitals, fantasize about having a kinship with the animal the toy represents, or cross over into plushy animal fetishes. You can tease and masturbate your lover with the toy, put on a show of masturbating with the toy yourself, or have a "threesome" with the stuffed animal. Also see "Furry Animal Costumes," above.

Tickling

Some might like to be tickled all over, have particular parts of their bodies (like feet) tickled, enjoy tickling someone who turns them on, like to watch sexy people tickle each other, or like tickling pushed to the limits with tears and involuntary urination. Many who like to be tickled become very aroused and will want to masturbate; you can restrain them and give them a hand job while you tickle them or employ any other devious scenario you think they might like—just tickle them while you do it. If they like to watch tickling, then put on a tickling video, employ dirty talk with role-playing tickling scenes, or momentarily tickle another person while your lover watches—then have hot sex while talking about it later. For a fun and sexy video featuring happy adult schoolgirls tickling each other to tears, see Maria Beatty's *Converted to Tickling*.

Wet and Messy, or Sploshing

Also called "WAM," this fetish is for seeing someone (usually attractive young women) soaked with water, covered in mud, or smeared with food—anything wet and messy, but the "splosher" will have their favorites. Some like to see fully clothed women at the moment of being hit with a burst of water, while others like to watch videos of girls pouring syrup, spraying whipped cream, and smearing cakes and pies all over their naked bodies. A messy fetishist also may want to masturbate while watching the action, have sex in the messiness, or get messy by themselves. A highly arousing photo collection of young women getting messy with food can be found in Charles Gatewood's *Messy Girls*. The premier messy magazine is *Splosh!* (woman-run website: www.splosh.co.uk). Find out about the messy community and more at www.messyfun.com.

Networking with Other Fetishists and Their Partners

Whether you want to find support from others in a similar relationship or get more ideas to make your fetish encounters erotically explosive, you can find cha-trooms, message boards, websites, and webrings (linked websites sharing a common theme) on the Internet dedicated to an astounding array of fetishes. If you don't have Web access it's a bit tougher to find community, but adult magazines found in porn shops cater to a myriad of fetishes, and in their back pages you'll find mail-order companies that carry a variety of fetish products and catalogs for more magazines, books, and videos.

But for fetishists and their lovers who have Internet connections, the world is your rubber-encased, spike-heeled, fetish oyster. As of this writing, the Web portal Yahoo! lists over 2,500 groups dedicated to fetish-related topics, with hundreds—sometimes thousands—of members in each group, all emailing, exchanging links, and communicating about their fetishes and their lives. Simply go to www.yahoo.com and click on "Groups," then type in the fetish group you'd like to connect with. Join one of the groups, and you'll have access to their message boards and links to more groups and resources dedicated to your fetish.

Other People's Panties

BY ALISON TYLER

Other people's panties turn me on. They always have. Ever since way back when… In college, whenever my pretty midwestern roommate was in class, I would dig through her lingerie drawer, fingering the seductive items she was saving to wear when her long-distance boyfriend was in town. Sometimes, I'd dress myself up in her favorite pieces: the matching leopard-print set she thought was particularly racy; or the black lace boy-cut shorts with a tank-style top. Other times, I'd just hold them to my naked body, caressing myself with the fine fabrics. I'd take my time to really smell the material before slipping on the garment, winning a whiff of laundry detergent, or perfume, lavender soap, or even the shadowy, lingering scent of real skin.

So I guess that's when it started. My fetish, I mean. Because at some point, wearing Lisa's clothing wasn't quite as important to me as sprawling on my tiny twin bed with the items in hand, stroking myself with the various intricate creations, coming while surrounded by panties and bras and camisoles that weren't mine. That was the key to my pleasure—the panties were someone else's, not purchased by me. Not meant for me. And the owner had no idea of my obsession with her private underthings. No idea at all.

By the end of the year, I had a set routine. Each day, I'd fondle the bikini bottoms Lisa carelessly discarded on the floor by her bed. I'd place them on my face and breathe in while I touched myself, reveling in the ghostly embrace of her, even though I didn't want her. I just wanted her knickers.

When the school year ended, my fetish remained. But I learned that I wasn't attached solely to Lisa's lingerie—*any* pretty woman's underthings would work. This is why I've never lived on my own, always have had a female roommate. I've worked to keep my desires hidden through years of flatmates, rifling undetected through laundry baskets, or top dresser drawers, or in the tangle of sheets at the bottom of a bed. My fantasies have deepened as I fingered the sweet-smelling satin hipsters, cotton bikinis, lace thongs. I have succeeded in getting my fill from my female roommates' collections, and I have never once told anyone about my fetish.

Not anyone.

Not even Jamie, my lover who swore on her heart that she'd love me through thick and thin, through sickness and health. I didn't tell her because our commitment ceremony included no line about loving through fetishes, through panty raids, through constant caressing with secreted sexy items. Although I planned to come clean at some point, I found that I couldn't confess. I told myself this was because I didn't know what she would say, didn't know how she might react to my treasured little secret. I pretended I simply couldn't bear to see disgust on her face.

Truthfully?

That wasn't it at all. I just didn't want to stop playing with her panties.

Jamie has perfect lingerie for my needs. She indulges herself in the finest fabrics, the prettiest panties in rainbows of colors. And though I can afford to buy myself the identical items, I know from experience that they wouldn't give me as great a pleasure as wearing Jamie's. Don't know why that is, but I can't change the fact. It's other people's panties that get to me.

If I'm in a pinch, I use a G-string or a thong snagged from the laundry basket, and I go for a quickie while Jamie thinks I'm taking a shower. But when my girlfriend is out for the evening, that's when I truly indulge. I make a whole night out of fucking myself with Jamie's underthings. First, I go through her dresser drawer, or our hamper, and pick out my pieces for the night. Sometimes I get off on a pair of her silky blue hipsters. I breathe in at the crotch. I run my tongue over the seam and taste her there. Or I use her cream-colored, lace-edged tap panties, which I love to watch her wear, but love even more to peel down her long, lean thighs. Occasionally, I dress myself up entirely in her naughty knickers, down to garters and stockings—but usually, it's enough to simply surround myself with an outfit or two, turning the mattress into a display fit for an underwear catalog, writhing around in all her lingerie, basking in the sea of her scent and her seductive taste.

This is all I've done, all I've ever needed—that is, until last night.

Jamie had plans to be out for the evening. As soon as I heard the front door close, I headed down to the bathroom. But this time, I found a surprise when I opened the hamper. Instead of her various clothing items strewn willy-nilly in the basket, they were neatly folded, with a red satin ribbon wrapping them up. I heard a noise behind me, and when I turned around, there was Jamie, waiting, a smile on her face. I didn't know what to say....

"I think they're your favorites," she said, grinning.

My hand fluttered over the blue satin, the soft pink lace, the black see-through thong.

"Yeah," I said, nodding. She was right.

"So take them out. Let me watch. I want to see what you do with them."

"How—" I started.

"Just do it, baby. I want to see."

Trembling, I took the bound package of my treasured items to the bedroom. Then I stripped and started. Jamie stood across the room, watching. At first, I was extremely aware of her staring at me, and I felt a prickle run through my body at the thought of being on display. But then I started to lose myself in the pleasure that always works through my body. I tuned everything out by focusing on the feel of the fabrics and the secret smell of Jamie's own scent embedded in her fine lingerie. I didn't even notice when she came closer and sat on the bed. Didn't tune into her until she finally moved right next to me, and she took the pieces from me and slowly rubbed them over my body. Everywhere I wanted her to.

And when I came, I whispered, "I didn't know you knew."

I looked at Jamie, into her lavender-blue eyes, at her flushed pink cheeks, and I saw how close she was to coming herself. This was as exciting for her as it was for me—I realized that in a heartbeat—the way she purred back at me. "It turned me on," she said, "when I figured out what you were doing. It made me wet to know that my panties made you wet...."

I guess sometimes you really don't know how another person feels...until you walk a mile—or fuck awhile—in their panties.

10

Erotic Dominance and Submission: S/M Fantasies

Dozens of books and videos explain in savory detail all the intricacies of rope tying, over-the-knee spanking, and how to choose a whip and wield it with menace on squirming submissives. But rather than tell you how to tie a knot or draw up a slave contract, I'd like to take you into the arousing realm of erotic dominance and submission fantasies—and let your imagination spark your desire for further study. You don't need to be a bondage whiz, a whip expert, or traditional S/M scenester, or know a famous dominatrix, to create hot fantasies that have a little—or a lot—of S/M in them. All you need is a motivation that turns you on and a little common sense about the practicalities. For learning the basics about ropes, whips, and scene negotiation, you'll find a complete list of books and videos in the Resources chapter.

These resources will open avenues of further study to you and help ensure that your journey into S/M is blissful, safe, and fun.

If you just flipped to this chapter, then flip yourself right back to Chapter 3, "Fantasies for Two," where you can read up on how to talk with your lover about what you do and don't want to try in the world of erotic fantasy. Fun and games with S/M that involve more than a decorative collar require that you both be honest and on the level about who does what to whom, and that you have an idea of how much, when, and how often.

If you have fantasies about being spanked, doing the spanking, being restrained by ropes, experiencing erotic embarrassment, giving power over to your lover, or taking total control of your loved one's every need (and satisfying a few of your own), your fantasy falls into the alluring realm of S/M. In these fantasies, one of you gives up control and the other assumes it. This arousing exchange generally involves captivity or bondage, and may involve punishment, erotic pain, or submission. Perhaps you will find both sides of the equation exciting, being both dominant and submissive. In the wonderful world of S/M, you can have your decadent cake and eat it—or be eaten—too.

Sweet Submission

A couple I know went to an S/M event where audience members could make charity donations to "buy" a slave for the evening. What this meant was that participants could bid on a contestant onstage who was either dominant or submissive; if they won, the person they "purchased" could choose to spend the evening with them. A very attractive young woman presented herself as a "love slave," and my excited friends bid on her—and won! However, when they got the young lady to a secluded spot in the club, they found that she wasn't sure what she really wanted. And neither were my friends. In the heat of the moment, the possibilities of bossing around a willing young gal had made them both horny and eager enough to land them in this fantasy-turned-predicament. As it turned out, they tied her up, tickled her a little bit, and then let her go. When they told me this story, I thought, *What a waste of resources!* The problem here is that both parties had fantasies about dominance and submission but neither had developed them beyond the point of "wouldn't that be fun."

When you want to give up control, a number of fantasy roles and scenarios can be tailored to the shape of your desires. Or roles may not even enter into it—you might be drawn to physical sensations rather than a role-based scenario. Perhaps you want physical restraint combined with sex or pain, or just a good, old-fashioned spanking. If you're purely a masochist, a person who is aroused or sexually pleased by receiving intense or painful stimulation, you may not necessarily be interested in power-exchange games where you "deserve" the punishment or submissively serve another person's needs. It may turn you on simply to have a gorgeous man or woman give you a long session of whipping, light strokes graduating to heavy flogging, releasing your endorphins and taking you to a state akin to a "runner's high." Or if restraint is your game, being completely tied down, or even "mummified" so that you cannot move a pinkie, might take you to new levels of arousal thanks to the feelings of helplessness—or comfort—that total restraint conveys.

But being submissive doesn't mean you have to be a masochist. You might get a thrill out of being a slave to your lover's every whim, from foot rubs to oral sex and more. You can be the silent handmaiden administering to his or her every need, in any costume or dramatic role you like, or you can be the sex toy that gets used and discarded—until you're needed for further use, that is. You can be ever-obedient in collar and slave attire, or you might enjoy being subtly owned by your lover, made to go *sans* panties in public, while in private you become your sweetie's serviceable love doll in garters and lace.

You don't have to misbehave to get spanked, and you don't have to be a slave to be sexually used by someone you love, but then again, if you do, you have a myriad of options for costumes and situations (see Chapter 4, "Role Play," for oodles of ideas). And it's important to note that while some people prefer submissive play in power-exchange fantasies, and others prefer to be dominant in every exchange, many people enjoy a bit of both worlds. Chances are, bits and pieces of what I mentioned above tickled your fancy here and there, bits that you can arrange to suit your fantasies about control. Who do you want to be?

A Sampling of Submissive Roles

Slave, submissive (as yourself or your real-life work role), secretary, maid, butler, schoolgirl/boy, criminal, cheerleader, nurse, victim, patient, military subordinate, prostitute, masseuse, altar boy/girl, housewife, unsuspecting husband, groupie, "innocent" passerby, human pet (pony, dog, cat), opposite gender.

Just as submissive roles lend themselves easily to spankings, punishments, humiliations, whippings, and more, dominant roles that become submissive—such as the haughty librarian being punished—make for red-hot fantasies. Don't let the classic stereotypes limit your imagination!

What happens to submissives? All manner of delicious predicaments. You may be required to serve your dominant—or a dominant couple—in a variety of ways. Read Chapter 6 to learn how to give an erotic striptease, lap dance, and erotic massage—which may come in handy if you are to give your dominant body service. Body services might include foot massages, grooming such as manicure and pedicure, facials, hair washing, drawing a bath and sensuously bathing your dominant, foot washing, towel-drying, full-body massage, erotic massage, sexual receptiveness, and oral sex. You might also be told to worship body parts or items that are important to your dominant—often features or objects that excite you, if your dominant is rewarding you. Follow your lover's instructions, which usually means kissing and nuzzling (or licking and fellating) feet, shoes, hands, whips, dildos, breasts, butts, genitals, panties, or other fetish items.

Domestic service might be for you. Submissive domestic service usually requires a costume or significant item of dress that says you're a servant. Maid or butler outfits can be practical, traditional, formal, or ridiculously sexy. Or you may have to scrub floors totally nude, or wearing only high heels and lipstick, kneepads and an apron, or in bondage. When you are a domestic, you might be expected to clean house, prepare meals, do laundry, and any other household chores that make you look sexy and vulnerable—and you will be expected to actually do the chores. If you are told to clean and condition the whips, you'd better do it! Don't perform a chore improperly in hopes of punishment. Also, expect to be interrupted during your chores (this is the fun part) for possible punishment and sexual services.

When Being in Charge Turns You On

When you read the story about the couple who "bought" a beautiful and willing submissive but had no idea what to do with her—did you find yourself thinking of a few things you might have done in their place? If you are typically dominant in your sex-play roles, or find yourself turned on by the thought of being in change, you're suited for the role of the dominant partner in a power-exchange dynamic. Dominants experience the heady rush of erotic power, the control, the responsibility for the submissive's pleasure and safety, and the mastery over S/M skills.

Being in control offers you a variety of personas, roles, and guises to choose from, all complementary to the role of your submissive. You may find yourself drawn to being in charge of a sexual interaction, calling the shots step by step. Or you might be a dominant who likes verbal and psychological control, ordering your lover to perform for you, rub your feet, give you head, or bend over. This mode of dominance, which works without pain or physical punishment, lends itself easily to character-driven role play, where you play boss to a secretary, teacher to student, sergeant to cadet, and so on. The scenes can be steamy and complex when you play authority figures who demand compromising sexual favors from whoever's in the submissive role—imagine the possibilities of babysitter and teenager, sleazy pornographer and starlet.

Does the title Master or Mistress suit you? Your power may extend further than in other roles you play, especially if you find the idea of punishing errant submissives exciting. As Master or Mistress, you may want to treat your submissive as owned property, inflict pain, use punishment as a behavioral tool, and be the absolute authority in your shared scenarios. As a newcomer in this role, you'll want to learn techniques for bondage and discipline, rope and whip techniques, and further study into negotiation and scene dynamics. The title "Master" or "Mistress" may be all you need to send you on your merry way, but if your shared tastes cry out for realistic techniques of punishment and control, please, do your homework.

If you're interested in sensation rather than psychology, you might like to assume the role of "top." The top doles out the whippings and spankings to the "bottom," but doesn't necessarily hold power over them. If your lover gets hot over the sensations of pain and pleasure but is turned off by the idea of being a submissive, you're the top and nothing more. If the person you're playing with simply enjoys pain and is not submissive, your function is to wield the whip—not to wield authority, punish bad behavior, or own the bottom as slave or property.

All these modes of being in charge are fluid, much like our sexual desires. You don't have to like doling out pain to be a stern and loving Mistress, and you might like the idea of paddling your lover but find authority figures too forbidding for you to portray. Put together a few or many of the elements I've suggested to craft the style of dominance that turns you on the most.

When it comes to power-exchange role play, you can establish roles and keep them throughout the scenario or create a scene that includes a dramatic moment when the tables are turned and the submissive becomes the dominant.

This scenario is a creative way to keep everyone happy in the case of a partner who wants a spanking but doesn't like submissive roles. A woman who loves to play the dominant but knows her boyfriend doesn't want to play the submissive can devise a scene in which she "flips" him. For example, he can begin by playing the stern teacher to her willful schoolgirl who defies his authority and gives him what he's got coming. Fun for everyone!

It's the job of the dominant to run the show according to everyone's wishes, and that includes cranking up the sexual heat. The dominant creates the predicament and dishes out the pain, pleasure, fear, embarrassment and desire, as he or she wishes. Dominants restrain, punish, and demand deeds such as housecleaning and body worship. They also show affection, which can relax a lover into trust and surrender and mixes nicely with power play. Doms keep the communication going; even if it seems one way, it's important to stay connected and keep the submissive excited by using dialogue to maintain the dramatic premise of the situation. It's also

A Sampling of Dominant Roles

Yourself (in daily life or your role at work), Master, Mistress, dominatrix, boss, teacher, headmistress, general, femme fatale, criminal mastermind, corporate CEO, policeman, FBI agent, kidnapper, jailer, animal trainer, doctor, nurse, sleazy pornographer, babysitter, older sibling, daddy or mommy, biker, football captain, coach, pimp, clergyman, rock star, producer.

important to maintain physical touch, whether a caress or a firm grasp—after all, this is a sensual experience. And doms know how to establish mood and atmosphere with clothing, candlelight, music, appropriate props, fetish items, and any other features that define the play-space. You can let your submissive see your toys before-hand to work up some anticipation, and even include toys more devious than those you intend to use to ratchet up the thrill. Have snacks and refreshments ready for afterward, when you're all spent and rosy-cheeked smiles.

Should you both decide to extend your S/M adventures outside the bedroom, there are a number of fun things you can do. Take a field trip—to Alcatraz, a torture museum, a dark cave, creepy mansion, or haunted house. Stray away from the tour if you get a chance, and menace your lover accordingly. Have your lover wear something that reminds them of their submission or connection to you—a decorative collar, leather under-wear, your underwear, no underwear, a rope under their clothing (anything that will go unnoticed by others).

You can make your submissive call you to ask permission for certain things, like what and when they can eat (be specific in your instructions), whether they can pee, what to wear, or how and when to masturbate. Exerting dominance while you're apart can be a nice prelude to a planned fantasy encounter, and if you go out together, you can take every opportunity to whisper what you're going to do to them later.

Captivity and Erotic Torment

Erotic captivity—bondage and erotic conquest fantasies—is one of the most common adult sexual fantasies. Confinement, servitude, and subjection all belong to captivity scenarios. Bondage, submission, and being on the receiving end of what the dominant dishes out are the most popular items on the menu. Most of these scenarios involve sex in some form, and you may decide whether or not your scenario involves force or coercion. The partner who is in charge might be doing it for the submissive's "own good," as therapy, or it might be a matter of force, "making" the submissive comply.

Captivity can be verbal or physical. Verbal confinement makes for complex and subtle levels of dominance and submission, and if you're the dominant you can whisper, demand, or command your submissive to do as they're told. You can tell them to hold still, pretend that they have on restraints, tell them to strip and put on a show, make them get into sexual positions, have them act as human furniture, compel them to hold objects while you have your way with them (schoolgirls can balance books on their heads), and punish them accordingly if they move, spill the glass of water, or otherwise disobey. You can also role-play holding them against their will, as in an espionage scenario.

Always Have a Safe Word

A safe word is a word that you both agree means "stop now." Pick an unusual word that you seldom use, and avoid using "no" or "stop" in case you'd like to be able to feign resistance to your predicament. Everyone who plays with captivity should have a safe word—some people have a word for "stop" and a separate word for "a little less, thank you." Stoplight colors—red, yellow, and green—are very popular. If one of you uses the safe word, stop the scene and switch to other activities.

When the captivity is physical, you'll be using real—not imaginary—ropes, metal handcuffs, leather cuffs, chains, or other items suitable for restraint. You can while away your time, erotically teasing and tormenting your lover as they lie tied to the bed, to themselves, to a chair, cuffed, restrained spread-eagled, or anything else you can cook up. Role-playing scenarios will present creative possibilities, such as medical fantasies involving bandages, jail fantasies with bars and cages, animal scenes with collars, harnesses and leashes, and Martha Stewart fantasies involving plastic wrap. Do keep medical scissors handy in case your knots are too tight, your bondage is painful or cuts off circulation, or your lover needs to get out of their restraints, fast. Do tie a long, colorful ribbon to your handcuff key so it's impossible to lose. Don't rest anyone's weight on bound or cuffed joints, and never tie anything around the throat, ever. If you gag your sweetie, establish a nonverbal safe word such as a gesture. Watch for jaw cramp, and be careful not to put too much in their mouth, which can cause a gag reflex. And remember—if you restrain them in public, you could attract the attention of the police and wind up in handcuffs yourself.

Teasing Your Captive

When you have your lover all tied up, here are a few suggestions of things you can do:

- Strip or masturbate just out of reach.
- Tell them how helpless and vulnerable they are. And all the things you might (and will) do to them.

- Rub their body slowly with fur, feathers, silk, satin, scratchy wool, panties, whips, or any fetish objects.
- Give them an erotic massage.
- Bite and scratch, spank and slap (not the face or testicles).
- Blindfold them—it's a great way to keep them guessing.
- Have your way with them sexually—very slowly, or rough and quick.
- Try hot and cold sensations. Rub them down with ice cubes or warm tea bags, or suck on an ice cube and then lick them with your cold tongue. Never put ice inside anyone's vagina or anus.
- Drip hot wax on them.
- Alternate pleasurable pain with genital stimulation.
- Apply clamps and clips to their body—but don't leave them on for more than five minutes. (Buy them in a specialty S/M store.)
- If tickling arouses them, have at it.
- Oral sex—giving or receiving. Face-sitting is nice, too.
- Shave their genitals.
- Use sex toys on them.

Pleasurable Pain and Punishment

Sometimes you must punish your submissive as part of training, and sometimes you catch them doing something really naughty... At these times, you'll need to discipline the bad boy or girl with something deliciously painful, "make" them accept their punishment, and if you want a cherry on top—"force" sexual favors. Don't forget—adults misbehave all the time. Pain isn't always a punishment, however; for some, it's the reward.

If punishment fits your scene, with intense sensations like clamps, spanking, whipping, paddling, and other types of pain, follow these guidelines and suggestions:

- It is absolutely required that you carefully discuss what is going to happen. It must be clear that you both want to explore pain in the context of erotic play. The receiving partner must give explicit consent.
- Start slowly; don't ratchet up the pain level before the recipient is suitably warmed up.
- Begin with light sensation. Your hands are ideal for this—caress, squeeze, knead, lightly slap, and spank.
- Speak to your partner throughout. You can speak in character, whisper dirty talk, and say things you know will excite your lover. Asking how they like what you're doing can be part of your dialogue.
- Alternate spanking or whipping with different tactile sensations such as fur, satin, heat, ice, hot wax, biting, and scratching.
- Never strike the lower back, head, neck, face, or bony areas such as the spine or knees.
- Stimulate your partner genitally.
- Don't forget to have fun incorporating bondage and blindfolds.
- Use sex toys.
- In a sixty-nine position, you can spank or penetrate them while they perform oral sex on you.

Public S/M Clubs

If you live in a large city, your kinky play needn't be confined to the privacy of your home. With nearly half of the adult population in the U.S. engaging in one form of kinky sex or another (according to Dr. Gloria Brame's book *Come Hither)*, and with the increasing acceptance of S/M imagery in the mainstream culture, more and more couples are becoming interested in and involved with S/M. Hence the proliferation of public S/M clubs and kinky-themed parties.

Public S/M dungeons are typically giant warehouses or dance clubs converted into a variety of themed play-spaces, with accommodations ranging from the mini-mal—a large room with some bondage equipment—to the outrageous. You're likely to see equipment that looks like movie set dressing: cages, racks, crosses, whipping benches, bondage chairs, and more. The larger, fully equipped clubs, such as San Francisco's Power Exchange, might have three levels, a dance floor, stripper pole, re-created jail cells, a decked-out dun-geon, and over a dozen themed rooms to satisfy almost any kind of fantasy play you can imagine. These bigger spaces also boast a number of areas where people can be publicly whipped and flogged, and professional dominants of all genders often make an appearance for public beatings of anyone who will make a donation to charity. These are the clubs where events such as slave auctions are held, often with theme nights such as "naughty schoolgirl" or military dress. If these clubs sound erotically interesting to you, get a little background and a primer for sex club etiquette in Chapter 8, "Public Sex."

Sex is seldom allowed in public S/M clubs, but when it is, safer-sex guidelines are required—condoms for all penetration, sometimes including fellatio. Because the clubs are open to the public, and even though most clubs make it expensive or prohibitive for single men to attend, single guys do turn up to watch couples and dominatrixes play, often masturbating while they watch. Couples or singles who want to avoid intrusive single men might choose to attend on couples-only nights, or take their play into more private spaces. The public clubs often have women-only and men-only nights as well. But for many, the thrill comes with being seen. Just the knowledge that someone is watching them administer a flogging or receiving a spanking is an incredible turn-on.

Public clubs generally advertise in the back sections of weekly newspapers—unless it's Halloween, of course, at which time these clubs may boast full-page ads in the main parts of the paper. You can also find them regionally through online sex resources such as www.Erosguide.com, www.Janesguide.com, and sex tourism books such as the *Horny?* guidebook series.

Check to see if there is a theme on the night you want to visit, or if there are limitations on attendees—no single men on certain nights, couples-only on Fridays, etc. Typically, the clubs impose strict dress codes, meaning no street clothes or business suits, and S/M gear, role-play costume, or fetish wear is required. A clothes check or lockers are provided to facilitate sexy dress. Admission prices vary, but on average you can expect to pay around $40 (and up to $75) per couple, about the same price for single men, and half that price for single women. Some clubs offer discounts for couples who provide a valid NASCA membership card (see Chapter 8, "Public Sex," for information on the North American Swing Club Association). Two women usually can get the couple's rate, and single men may have to agree to further restrictions such as wearing a towel, with very strict enforcement of the "no street clothes" rule. No drugs or alcohol are allowed in the clubs, and as with any sex party, don't bring unneeded valuables with you into the club.

Organizations and Private Clubs

There are BDSM organizations in all major North American and European cities, populated by beginners, dabblers, regular players, professionals, and lifestyle players. These organizations provide a place for the local community to network, socialize, learn from each other, work on projects together, and create private events where members can play in fully equipped private dungeons. You don't need to be a member of any club to enjoy and learn about BDSM, nor do you need to join just to see their listings of private playspaces. Quite a few S/M organizations organize play parties for their members only, but you can also find parties open to nonmembers; these organizations often publish a calendar of events. They can open a window to worlds you might find exciting to explore, provide referrals to reputable professional doms, and give you access to private playspaces where strict etiquette protects you from interlopers interrupting your scene, or thumping dance music ruining your prison-cell fantasy.

Kinky and S/M subcultures may seem shrouded in mystery, rife with odd rules, signals, and customs, and punctuated with jargon and code words. But educational and support groups for members are warm and welcoming to newcomers, and their calendars include everything from casual meetings to demonstrations of various techniques and special-occasion parties. These subcultures' S/M play parties and events will be a far cry from the wild party scene of public S/M clubs; in its place you'll find a group that takes its S/M play and behavioral rules very seriously *and* knows how to have a wickedly hot time. Events featuring S/M play include dungeon evenings, charity fund-raisers, leather fairs, and street festivals. Be prepared to see things at these events you've never seen before, and to soak up a lot of kinky inspiration.

Seeing a Professional Dominatrix

Have you ever wanted to turn over control to an experienced, professional dominant woman or man? A dominatrix (also called a *domme*, or *dom*) might fit the bill. With a pro, you can taste the experience of submission—or share dominance—with a tried-and-true expert. You can watch your lover being bound and disciplined, you can take turns, or you can negotiate any type of power-exchange fantasy you have in mind.

Whether you're both just a little interested in playing kinky games or are well-versed in S/M scenes and power play, a session with a professional dominatrix, BDSM instructor, or professional male dominant can spice up your sex play and leave you with wonderfully wicked ideas to explore on your own. Pro doms have years of experience, all the equipment you can imagine, and dungeons and fantasy playrooms where they can make your power-exchange fantasies come true. And, while seeing a pro dom means that there is no sexual contact of any kind, you can bet you won't be able to keep your hands off each other after leaving the sexually supercharged atmosphere of the dungeon.

With a pro dom, you can safely explore fantasies such as being tied up, spanking, whipping, punishment, bondage in leather or ropes, role-play scenes that involve dominance and submission, foot worship, transvestitism, and even fetish fantasies that include rubber, isolation, human animal play, adult babies, mummification, and other exotic pursuits. Some dominants and commercial dungeons also offer fantasy sessions that are not necessarily S/M in nature. You can negotiate a scene where one of you experiences one of these scenarios while the other watches; where you both submit together; you both take turns submitting; one "assists" the dominant; or one of you is tied up and "forced" to watch. As long as there is an exchange of power where one or both of you is submissive, the sky's the limit. A number of dominatrixes specialize in doing scenes with couples, and some offer tutoring sessions in dominance training.

Discuss with your partner beforehand what you'd like to get out of a scene. Will either of you want to submit, watch, or assist? Do you want to trade off, or try submission after watching first? You're going to need to discuss specifics when you negotiate the scene with the dominant; the more details you have worked out, the more satisfying you can make your scene. Reputable dominants who work on their own offer telephone consultations in which you discuss your fantasies, the dominant's limits, and your limits, and make decisions about scenarios. When you call a commercial dungeon that employs multiple dominants, you will speak to a fantasy consultant who will direct you to the professional who can best bring your scene to life. Or you may be asked to come in to negotiate in person, and you may be given a tour of the facilities (the address is typically disclosed once you make an appointment). Discretion and privacy are given priority in every exchange. Some use the term *couple* interchangeably with *group*, so when you call you may hear about "group" rates (or "donation" rates, depending on the local laws). Be sure to select a dominatrix or dungeon that explicitly states they do sessions with couples.

Seeing a dominatrix or visiting a commercial dungeon isn't cheap—but it can be an experience well worth saving up for. Sessions are typically booked for half-hour or one-hour time slots. You can expect base prices at a commercial dungeon to start at $100 for a half-hour session and $140 for a full hour, and high-priced dungeons will charge as much as $1000 an hour. Individual dominants may charge $200 per hour. Ask what types of payment they accept before you arrive—commercial spaces accept credit cards and cash, as do most private practitioners—and be sure to ask what name will appear on your billing statement if you have privacy concerns. Payment is made before your session.

11

Sex Games

How far are you prepared to go in your quest for erotic fun? Sex games are for adventurous lovers who are willing to try something new on a dare, like smearing each other with whipped cream, taking naughty photos, making their own dirty movies, and using Internet technology to share live webcams of their most exposed moments.

Ten Erotic Escapades

Maybe it's that when we get turned on, our minds become a little bit devious. Take seduction and arousal as far as it can go with a simple sex game—a little tip, trick, or suggestion to spice up your routine or make your sexual encounter unforgettable.

Fit to Be Tied

Tie your lover's hands together and then invite them to make love to you. Watch them trying to remove your undies with their teeth. Next time, switch roles.

Treasure Hunt

Leave a series of notes and sexy presents like sex toys and batteries, lube and champagne, leading your lover throughout the house until they reach the final prize—you.

Sex Coupons

Make your own redeemable sex coupons, and present them as a package, present them as "rewards," or hide them one at a time where your lover will find them. Make them redeemable upon receipt, and good for things like "a quickie," "hot oral sex," and "role play as an erotic masseuse."

Daring-Do

Trade erotic dares, seeing how far you will go. Dare your lover to tell you a fantasy, a sexual secret, perform a striptease, masturbate, flash you in public.

The Voyeur

Give your lover permission to watch you from a secret hiding place as you undress and bathe—then crank up the heat by masturbating. Make sure to put on a really good show.

Any Game Will Do

Play any game—miniature golf, poker, pinball, pool—with the prize being that the winner's erotic fantasy comes true. In a twist on this game, the loser gets tied up, spanked, or must put on a dirty show.

Show and Tell

Tell your lover which parts of his or her body really turn you on, and why. Touch the hot spots as you talk about them. Take turns.

Sex Mannequin

One of you becomes a mannequin, unable to move while you are being touched, kissed, undressed, fondled, and especially, penetrated. Next time, switch.

Shopping Spree

Buy your sweetie a gift certificate to an adult sex toy store and set an expiration date—make the date an upcoming weekend at a hotel.

Video Captive

Rent or buy an X-rated video and watch it together—but make it a rule that while you can touch your partner, they must keep their hands to themselves. Trade roles after each sex scene.

Messy Fun

Maybe you're not the type to play with your food, but you might change your mind after you see what happens when you turn your lover into a squirming, giggling—and horny—dessert. A spoonful of warmed chocolate sauce drizzled over a pair of sensitive nipples feels like heaven, and it's a delicious aphrodisiac for whomever gets to lick it off. An affectionately restrained sweetheart can do little but enjoy the teasing and arousing torment you deliver with a bottle of raspberry syrup, sticky drips of honey, chilled whipped cream—and your hot mouth on the job for thorough cleanup. Better yet, two can play, painting each other with frosting, dousing each other in syrup, rubbing messy sweets all over each other.

There are a few important things to remember when playing with your food. Food, especially sweet and sugary foods, should be kept away from the vagina. Sugars can cause yeast infections, and oils are difficult to flush from the vaginal canal. Because latex—condoms, dental dams, gloves—break easily when exposed to oil, you'll need to be extra cautious playing with food and latex (see Chapter 12 for additional information on safer sex). And finally, never, ever squirt or spray anything (like whipped cream) or insert bottles into vaginal or anal openings.

Caressing him or her with juicy fruits or drips of honey is decadent and wonderful, and you can really spice things up if you incorporate aphrodisiacs into your edible seductions. Aphrodisiacs are foods and beverages that have been used historically to ignite the senses, seduce, and stir the passions of those who consume these romantic treats. In some cases, the herbs, fruits, or spices

Aphrodisiac Seductions

Leave the utensils in the kitchen and bring these stimulating treats to bed:

- Strawberries and chocolate sauce
- A salad of quartered figs, shredded basil, and drips of balsamic vinegar, but no fork
- Warmed honey and a spoon for drizzling
- Vanilla-bean ice cream, but no spoon
- Licorice or candied rose petals beside the bed as a snack
- Mango or papaya spears wrapped in mint leaves

stimulate the flow of blood to the genitals, heating up the lower body and increasing arousal. Ingest aphrodisiacs on an empty stomach to maximize their beneficial attributes, and don't fill up—you won't want to be too full to have sex! Here are a few wonderful aphrodisiacs for messy fun or finger food: avocados, basil, cinnamon, coffee, chocolate, damiana (an herb), fennel, figs, grapes, honey, lavender, licorice, mangoes, mint, oysters, papaya, rosemary, rose petals, strawberries, and vanilla.

Messy play can be—messy. Plan ahead for your messy adventures and use precautions so you don't have to have the carpet steam-cleaned or throw away your nice flannel sheets:

- For the really messy fun, set the scene in your bathtub or shower. If you get cold when you're all messy, douse yourselves with a jet of warm water.
- You can buy plastic tablecloths in a variety of colors and patterns, and at party supply stores you can buy rolls of colorful plastic sheeting. Put plastic down as a protective layer on your bed, the floor—wherever you want to play. If you don't like the feel of plastic under you, cover it with an old sheet.
- For mildly messy adventures, a few thirsty towels on the bed will do—though I'd advise against using light-colored towels.
- Have a few warm washcloths ready for spills—and for cleaning up what your mouth misses.

Ready, set...smear, drip, and taste! Here are a few lip-licking suggestions:

- Indulge in an after-hours feast. Feed each other finger foods and sexy treats such as grapes or strawberries, banana slices dipped in Nutella, or your fingers dipped in whipped cream and chocolate.

- With finger foods, "accidentally" smear a little on your lover's mouth and kiss it off.
- "Accidentally" smear food on the chin, nape of the neck, chest, nipples—or lower.
- Squeeze juice from fruits onto each other's skin, or crush them onto each other and eat them off.
- Tickle sensitive spots with cool fruits.
- Create mountain peaks of chocolate or whipped cream on nipples.
- Body-paint each other with different colors of frosting.
- Think about what foods will taste and smell good together. Sweet syrups and sauces are highly recommended, and you can find an array of colors and flavors at your supermarket.
- You don't have to limit yourselves to drippy sauces. Cream pies, cakes, pastries, and anything that is sweet and squishy can be smeared on breasts, squished on buttocks, or slathered onto a cock.
- All these suggestions go nicely with a blindfold, or when that sexy someone is all tied up. See Chapter 10.

So, You Want to Be in Pictures?

Sexual imagery has a powerful effect on us. An arousing image, in a photograph or onscreen, can take us from neutral into overdrive in seconds flat—sometimes completely by surprise. You've probably seen the effect on your lover of a sexy picture or scene in a movie; they may be momentarily transfixed, with a secret smile or sparkle in their eye and a secret fantasy running in their head. What if you were the star of their show?

You can easily produce your own erotic photographs, create adult videos as mementos of your hot encounters or as hot porn that turns you both on, or initiate steamy interactions by taking turns behind the camera. All you need is a camera, some uninterrupted time, and your erotic imagination. When you make your own erotic movies or images, you have a number of sexy options:

- Shoot or film each other undressing, bathing, rubbing on lotion, erotically shaving, or masturbating.
- With a tripod, photograph both of you doing anything that turns you on the most—undressing, making out, performing oral sex on each other, or having sex in any position.
- Enact a steamy role-playing scene (see Chapter 4, "Role Play"), someone's hottest fetish fantasy (see Chapter 9, "Fetishes"), or a riveting S/M encounter (see Chapter 10, "Erotic Dominance and Submission: S/M Fantasies").
- Create a scenario with a storyline, or reenact a scene from a movie you both find arousing. Layer in props, outfits, location, and shoot in the style of your favorite director or photographer.
- Different photos or videos can be created for different moods—for example, romantic, dreamy, playful, or hot and nasty.

Digital vs. Analog

When shooting erotic stills or video of yourselves, you have two options: using a digital camera or an old-fashioned analog film camera. Both have advantages and considerations for convenience, privacy, and ease of use.

Digital cameras can take dozens—hundreds—of pictures in one session, have become relatively inexpensive, and are easy to use. The screen allows you to compose your shots more easily than a standard small viewfinder hole; you can see the finished product immediately; and if you take a picture or shoot footage you don't like, you can delete it on the spot. The digital images can be downloaded onto your computer, where you can print stills, edit footage into a film, and send pictures or video to a lover.

Privacy can be an issue with digital stills and video. Keeping images on your computer is risky if anyone else shares your computer, and is not advised for work or family computers. Store your image or video files on a disk, stash the disk in a safe place, and remember to "empty" your system's trash. Be sure to delete the images from your camera and empty your computer's trash with the camera connected to your computer (to ensure that you wipe all the pictures off the camera). If you email the pictures, know that email can sometimes be intercepted: Your employer can legally read email sent from, to, or through your work email address. Also, most mail programs save mail in a "sent" folder, which you will want to delete.

But most importantly, with digital images, take and share explicit erotic images only with people you absolutely trust. If your relationship is on the rocks, you're trying to patch a breakup, you're having an affair with someone who is attached or married, or if your relationship isn't permanent, you risk giving digital erotic images to people who can post them, send them to others, or do a number of compromising things with them on the Internet. It takes less than an hour and a basic skill set to set up a primitive website. Know your partner well, and have a history of trust established between you.

Film cameras, whether stills or videotape, bring their own considerations, plusses, and minuses. On the minus side, two drawbacks are readily apparent: You cannot send a 5 x 7 photo instantly via email (though it can be scanned as a digital image), and if someone stumbles across your pictures or VHS cassette, you're instantly busted. On the plus side, film images have a warmer quality than digital, and (at least for the present) they look better printed and the prints are much more affordable. Film cameras also have become relatively inexpensive, though for stills you'll have to get your film developed somewhere—and you don't want to end up on some employee's personal "wall of fame." For confidentiality and safety with stills, use a Polaroid or other instant camera. Polaroids make a very sexy token of a hot encounter.

The final disadvantage of analog film and video is that you can't edit on the fly as you can with a digital camera, which is tailor-made for changes and instant deletions. Some couples like to exploit this "unforgiving" aspect of the analog medium, and consider its spontaneity and its ability to unflinchingly capture the moment— no matter how compromising—an asset.

Erotic Video and Photo Basics

To create a successful sequence of sexy photos or an erotic video, keep in mind the following suggestions:

- Have your location, costumes, sex toys, and props ready.
- If you have a story or script, think it through. Get a pen and paper, and sketch your shots—you don't have to be an artist; use stick figures!
- Decide on your lighting style before you begin— dark and romantic, eloquent and warmly lit, natural and with outside light (can be reflected using white sheets or paper), or glossy and well lit.

- Try to take test shots or footage before you begin.
- Whoever ends up in front of the camera should face at least one-third toward the camera, or you'll miss capturing the action in your camera's frame.
- Choose a variety of shots: wide shots that capture the whole room, medium shots that frame the body, close-ups that crop everything except faces or the focus of the action, extreme close-ups of mouths, breasts, genitals.
- The farther away you are from your subject, the shakier your image.
- Avoid too many wide shots, or you'll yearn for more detail later.
- Decide on the camera's point of view. Is it a fixed position, like a tripod, or movable, like a person? Whose point of view does it represent—yours, your lover's, or another person's?
- Always shoot what turns you on.

Make Your Own Porn

Have you ever seen a porn video and thought you could do it better? You can. Want to make a sexy movie of yourselves to watch and get inspired by? It's easy. Do you want to hold the camera and direct your lover to orgasm, or put on a private show yourself? Grab a video camera and get started.

Video cameras come in an array of formats, but you'll most likely be using VHS, Video 8, High 8, digital 8, or Mini DV. Each type is as easy to operate as a point-and-shoot camera but also offers complex options for investigating advanced camera techniques. Two things these cameras do on their own are autofocus and light balance; to get clear shots you'll want to adjust your camera movements around these functions.

Practice first to see how the camera reacts to focus and light changes. Always move (pan) the camera slowly to give it time to focus, and the same goes for zooming in or out. Should you want to move closer, first make sure the lens is zoomed out to its widest setting. If the light is coming from behind your subject, focus or zoom in on them to reduce the background light source in the frame—otherwise they will look like dark silhouettes.

A tripod not only frees you up to enter the shot and join your lover, but also provides a reliably solid base to keep the camera steady. Many higher-end digital video cameras have a steady-correction system that reduces shakiness, but no shot will be steadier than the hand that holds the camera. If you like the idea of hand-held shots and the first-person realism they convey, try to shoot using both hands, keeping your arms tucked against your body for stability. Leaning against a wall, doorframe, or other stable object will help, as will standing with your feet apart, sitting, propping your elbows on a table, or lying across an ottoman or on your stomach.

Sound is important. As a porn reviewer, I've had my libido crushed, trampled, and seen it run for the hills by many a porn film with wretched sound or ridiculous music. The mistakes made by many "professional" porn auteurs are easy to avoid. First of all, have your subjects make noise—dirty talk, panting, groaning, whatever is authentic and arousing. Next, be aware of your background noises—they can make or break a scene. The sound of traffic outside can enhance an urban, city-dwelling setting, but the sound of kids playing on your neighbor's lawn can ruin everything. Decide if you want music—it's often unnecessary and a distraction. Avoid having your music coming from a stereo or other source in the room, which sounds like crap in the final video; instead, add the music afterward as a subtle layer.

Your Erotic Photo Shoot

Most erotic photographers I've worked with and interviewed for this book prefer 35 mm cameras. SLR (single lens reflex) cameras are pricier than others, but turn out great shots and show the photographer just what the shot will look like through the viewfinder. But you don't have to break the bank to get breathtaking photos—even 35 mm disposable cameras available at drugstores and supermarkets can yield great shots. Wacky toy cameras can make for artful, sexy, and fun shoots as well, and tend to be inexpensive. In general, Fuji film brings more greens and blues to finished pictures than Kodak film, which produces heavier reds and yellows. When shooting erotic photos with film rather than with a digital camera, you'll need to do your own developing or have them developed by a trusted friend. Instant Polaroid cameras circumvent developing issues but lack quality—though you can buy close-up lenses and black-and-white film to make your erotic Polaroid photos more exciting.

Digital cameras are easy to use, fun to edit and manipulate, ensure privacy with at-home printing, enable you to email or post pictures via the Internet, and they provide instant gratification. You can find disposable digital cameras in drugstores for a pittance, or you can invest in high-resolution cameras with oodles of effects, on-board video, and professional lenses. Read the section above, "Make Your Own Porn," for tips on keeping your camera steady, autofocus, and automatic light balance. With a digital camera, take into account the one-second lag time from pressing the button to taking the actual shot.

Set up your studio, and you're ready to go! Consider your background, avoiding busy patterns that will distract from your subject. If you're shooting in public, see Chapter 8, "Public Sex," for tips on safety. Hang a bedsheet or a roll of colored paper, position your lover in front of a wall, or on a bed with few conflicting patterns. Gather a variety of fun props and sex toys—you'll try many different props and positions as you go along. Expect to take a lot of pictures to end up with a few good ones—that's how the pros do it. Play around with what the camera sees by experimenting with anonymous close-ups, having your subject look at you directly, just past you, or away from you, and try different expressions. Provoke your subject with questions and comments—make them laugh, snarl, seduce, or melt for the camera.

Cybersex

We are wired for sex. Our brains drive us to seduce, tease, arouse, and to be led by desire and erotic passion—so it's no wonder we've adapted sexually so very well to the Internet. Even those who know little about JavaScript and think the only use for a router is to cut wood have learned to make email salacious, chatrooms into virtual sex clubs, and webcams into peep booths. We are millions of dirty-minded primates with millions of high-tech typewriters to play with.

Cybersex is a blanket term for sexually explicit exchanges using Internet technology, including email, instant messaging, chatrooms, digital cameras, and transfers of audio and image files. Cybersex also refers directly to the act of sex with another person while you are both online via instant messaging or in a chatroom, talking dirty to each other, scene-building, possibly role-playing, and masturbating. You'll see the word used as a synonym for the word *fuck*, typically *cybering* or, as a noun, *cyber*. Using Web technology for sex has made communication with faraway lovers both afford-able and thrilling, and has made connecting sexually with strangers more exciting than ever. On the Web, you can be yourself or someone you've always wanted to be, and can communicate with people you'll never see (unless you want to). It's private, it's anonymous, and you can try any sexual fantasy imaginable. The Web has freed our culture sexually in ways we have yet to discern.

Email

Email is probably the easiest and most convenient tool for cybersex. You can write a naughty note, compose a dirty letter, or jot down a raunchy suggestion—all you have to do is press "send" and it's in your lover's mail-box instantly. And unlike the phone or chatrooms, it allows you to take your time composing your message.

A sexy email can be as simple as a note saying that you're having a fantasy about your partner, telling them what you want to do to them later, or composing an erotic short story about the two of you. I once sent a cybersex lover a fantasy about meeting in person—but I sent it a few paragraphs at a time, over the course of a few days. I don't consider myself an erotica writer; I simply wrote what I knew turned both of us on. You don't need to be a writer at all to send them sexy sto-ries—instead, send them a link to a hot story you found on a website. If you're planning an S/M encounter, you can send your sweetie suggestive emails to get them excited about the encounter to come—for example, telling them you want them completely shaved, or you want to come home and find them ready for whatever you have in mind. Sending erotic photos, short videos, or voice recordings as file attachments is also fun.

Be very careful about sending erotic emails using computers at work, or sending them to lovers while they're at work. Companies can legally monitor employees' email sent from work, whether anonymous or not, and can fire you for sending sexually suggestive emails. One way to get around this might be to use personal wireless handheld computers, PDAs, or cell phones to send text messages, which should be fine if none of it is paid for by your employer. Don't ever install software on work computers for your adult fun and games, as some services that do more than email, such as text messaging and instant messaging, might require.

Text Messages and Instant Messaging

Text and instant messages are like sending email, except whoever you're sending to can respond instantly, so the two of you can have a conversation—between computers, from computers to phones, between phones, with wireless PDAs such as Palm or Sony Clié, or with other devices like "hip-tops" and pagers. You can use any device capable of receiving a text message, and you don't have to worry about long distance charges if you're sharing text phone sex with someone far away. For tips on phone sex and talking dirty, read Chapter 6, "Weaving a Spell."

Online, you can find several free services that will allow you to download what you need for messaging. Yahoo! Messenger, AOL Instant Messenger (AIM), ICQ, and Instant Messenger are popular. Try to make sure your lover isn't at work or in a compromising place when they receive your message, as some services chime to announce a new message, drawing attention from anyone nearby who might be able to see the computer screen. But once you start, unleash the dirty talk—you can direct your lover to masturbate, explicitly describe what you're doing to yourself, or engage in role-play fantasies. You may learn to type very well with one hand!

Chatrooms

From anywhere in the world, a person can log into a chatroom and communicate instantly with scores of people at once—as many as there are in the "room" at that moment. The messages are seen instantly by everyone in the room, and you can have group or solo conversations with total strangers, using any name, description, and role you like. You can arrange to meet cyber lovers in certain rooms for trysts. Chatrooms have possibly become the most popular places for meeting virtual sex partners and having anonymous sex.

You can find chatrooms on Yahoo!, www.iFriends.com, ICQ, and MSN Chat, to name a few, including services dedicated to gay men and lesbians, services that provide free chatrooms for anyone, and rooms divided into categories and subjects. Many sites like Yahoo! include staff- and user-created sections: The staff sections offer topics like knitting and antiques, but the-user created sections are where you find the sex rooms (carefully safeguarded from minors), with themes ranging from arousing to crass. Some services require that you download an application in order to chat.

Chatrooms are semipublic, so if you are even a little bit of an exhibitionist, you'll find yourself in heaven talking dirty and having anonymous sexual interactions with strangers while others can comment or just "watch." If showing off isn't necessarily your cup of tea, most services have options for creating a private room with another user in the form of a single pop-up text message window, where you can cyber together uninterrupted and unwatched. Some of the private rooms permit you to "enable voice" with your computer's microphone and speakers.

Because anyone can enter a chatroom, you may run into users who are rude, abusive, offensive, or just annoying. Remember that you are completely anonymous, and you are safe from all but a temporary irritation. Every service offers a menu option allowing you to block the messages of anyone else in the room. It's like erasing them from your screen room—you no longer see their messages. By the same token, anyone in your chatroom may assume any role or persona they please, so err on the side of caution when you choose to interact with anyone beyond the anonymity of the chatroom. Don't give out any personal information or offer further contact outside the room. It's just like meeting any stranger—be smart, safe, and cautious.

Webcams and Digital Images

Take an erotic digital picture of yourself, and you can send it attached to an email, a text message, or to someone in a chatroom. Many chatrooms allow you to connect a webcam so you can send real-time video to whomever you're cybering with. Camera phones have taken erotic spontaneity to the next level, giving users a toy to snap explicit photos anywhere, anytime, and send them as email or text attachments.

When snapping a digital image to send via email or text message, be sure your camera is set to the lowest resolution to avoid sending a giant file attachment that might clog up your lover's inbox. If a webcam sounds more your style, you'll find digital cameras that can double as a webcam—though webcams themselves are now relatively inexpensive. Mind you, with a webcam you're not sending a video transmission; instead, the images will come through in a broken stream about every three seconds or so. If you want a moving picture, you'll have to take short movies of yourself, save them as QuickTime files, and send them as attachments, just as you'd send a picture.

Show-and-Tell

BY ALISON TYLER

I know it's silly, but I like game-playing in the bedroom. Every once in a while, I read about romantic couples who require only a little candlelight and soft jazz in order to get in the mood. Sometimes I envy them. Sometimes I think they must be lying. Candlelight and mood music are fine—when you're going for ambiance at a fancy restaurant. But in the bedroom, what I need is that friction that only comes about for me when someone's willing to play kinky. To dress me up or tie me down. To talk dirty or use a blindfold. To break out the sex toys, the whipped cream, the handcuffs.... Or, my favorite, to play show-and-tell.

For me and Hank, show-and-tell is far different from the childhood activity of parading some new trinket in front of a room of bored classmates. For me and Hank, show-and-tell is a special sort of game, in which I show him more of myself, if he tells me something delicious that I don't know about him.

It starts like this: I dress up in something incredibly slinky—garters, marabou-trimmed nightie, high heels, gloves—the sorts of things that drive men crazy. Or, at least, *my* man crazy. Then I perch myself on the edge of my rose-pink vanity table, and I let Hank get a good long look at me. I wait until I know he's ready.

"All right," I say, finally. "You start."

He pretends to think about it, making me wait. He always makes me wait. Right when I start to squirm, he begins. "Once," he says, "I picked up a girl while I was on a date with someone else."

"Continue—" I say, as I start to slide one long velvet glove off.

"My date was in the restroom, and this hot young thing had been batting her eyes at me all night long, and I gave her my business card and a kiss at the bar."

"You scoundrel," I say.

"She'd left her number on my answering machine by the time I got home."

I fling him my glove and then perch again, waiting.

"Another time," he says, "I fucked a girl in a swimming pool."

"So?"

"At a hotel."

"And?"

"In the middle of the afternoon..."

"Yes...?"

"While sunbathers baked obliviously around us."

He wins my other glove for this story, and now that my hands are free, I start to touch myself through my panties while I wait for story number three. Or *snippet* number three, I should say. His memories are tiny flickers of pleasure. I like to hear them as much as he likes to watch me undress. I enjoy reliving his frisky fairy tales, and I picture Hank starring in every scene he describes.

Tonight, his stories tease me out of my negligee, out of my right shoe and stocking. I'm almost naked, and that makes me even more aroused. The waiting is intense— waiting to take everything off.

"There was this one girl who liked to fuck in public," he says.

"Really?"

"Start on that shoe," he admonishes me.

I bend my leg and slowly undo the buckle.

"She kept after me to let her come to my office."

"Yeah?" I have the buckle undone, but I take my time removing the high-heeled Mary Jane.

"When she finally slipped in at the end of a work day, we fucked on my desk all night long. I didn't even get to go home and shower before the workday started again."

I hand him the shoe, and he breathes in deep, savoring my scent, then motions for the stocking.

"You go first," I say.

"I had phone sex on an airplane."

"No kidding?"

"In first class, but all I could do was respond with yesses or nos. The compartment was packed and she tried her best to make me lose control. To make me forget where I was."

I give him my stocking and then wait, panties the last thing on. He's almost won, I guess. Or have I?

"I made a girl cry once," he says.

"Heartbreaker."

"No," he shakes his head, and I can see a light in his deep brown eyes. "She wanted me to."

"So spill it."

"So start pulling down those panties, baby."

I work my fingertips under the waistband as he says, "She needed a spanking, this girl. Man, did she need a spanking. She was that sort of a girl. The kind you want to bend over and paddle on sight. But she thought I was going to give her a little patty-cake-style punishment session. Light and sweet on her perfect, heart-shaped ass. That's what she thought, at least. But she didn't know me well enough. She didn't understand my true character."

I pull my panties down my thighs, down past my knees, and then I turn around and bend over at the waist so he can see everything. My fingertips are on the edge of my vanity, and I gaze at myself in the mirror as he continues his tale.

"I held her in place," he says, "and I spanked her bare bottom until she cried… and until she came."

I kick off the panties, and then stand and turn around, grinning at him as he reaches to snatch them up off the floor.

He's talking about me. But that's no big surprise. He was talking about me the whole time. I'm the girl he picked up on a date. The girl he fucked in a swimming pool. The one who tried to make him shoot in the first class cabin—Christ, was that fun! I'm the girl who screwed him on his desk all night long, and yes, I was the one he spanked to tears, and to orgasm.

They're all me.

They're *always* me.

But somehow when he tells and I show, I wind up learning more about him and more about me, every single time.

12

Safer Sex

When we have sexual adventures, we want our memories to be of hot sex, once-in-a-lifetime erotic peaks, and trying out decadent fantasies that would make Hollywood blush. We don't want those memories tainted by a hasty decision not to use a condom, a dental dam, or gloves—resulting in a sexually transmitted infection or virus. We have to care about ourselves and the people we have sexual contact with. We can start by practicing safer sex.

You might wonder why I employ the term *safer sex* instead of *safe* to indicate the practice of using barriers and proper lubrication to prevent injury and the spread of disease. That's because the use of barriers (such as condoms) is not a hundred percent foolproof in protecting against STDs. There are many factors involved in every sexual encounter: Each party assesses the risks in every situation, often making snap judgments in the heat of the moment. This is especially true when you're in a couple and trying out a threesome, sex parties, swinging, or having sex with strangers. The term *safer* means that safe-sex gear is safer than no protection at all.

Always use plenty of water-based lubricant, even if you don't think you need it. Sex feels incredible with slicked-up parts, and latex tends to absorb moisture, making condoms more susceptible to breakage. A drop of lube in the tip of a condom gives more pleasure and sensation to both the wearer and the recipient of penetration—once you try it, you'll never go back! Water-based lubes are friendly to the vaginal ecosystem, won't degrade latex (a tiny bit of oil will destroy latex almost instantly), and come in hypoallergenic formulas. Avoid lubes with Nonoxynol-9, which causes abrasions on mucous membranes, and sensitive women should avoid lubes with glycerin, a sugar that contributes to yeast infections.

The Gear

Before you put each other's naughty bits in your mouths or even think about rubbing your bodies together, it's a good idea to know where these bits have been. But since we don't live in a perfect world, you'll want to use condoms, gloves, dental dams, or finger cots when you have oral, vaginal, and anal sex—and in some cases, when you give hand jobs. When your partner pulls out a condom, dam, glove, or cot, you know you're in good hands. See Chapter 13, "Resources," for places to get all kinds of safer-sex gear. The following items are your first lines of defense against infections and viruses:

Condoms

A condom is a snug sheath that unrolls onto a penis or sex toy. They are available in latex, polyurethane, and animal skin, in dozens of sizes, colors, and flavors. Use condoms for fellatio, vaginal and anal sex, and for covering sex toys that are made of porous materials, or when you want to share a sex toy. Change condoms for different sex partners and orifices—anything used anally should be covered with a condom before being inserted orally or vaginally. Do not use oils of any kind where latex condoms may come in contact; polyurethane condoms may be used with oils. Animal-skin condoms do not prevent the spread of some viruses.

Dental Dams

These are thin squares of latex or polyurethane used as a barrier for cunnilingus and rimming. Lubricate the genitals, place the dam on top, keep a good hold on the dam, and lick to your heart's content. Available in a few flavors and colors, and in a pinch you can use plastic wrap or a condom cut open and laid flat.

Gloves

Use latex or nonlatex gloves for hand jobs on any gender. They protect the genitals from germs carried on your hands, can protect your hands from picking up viruses or germs, and make hands a smooth surface free of jagged nails or scratchy calluses.

Finger Cots

Tiny condoms made of latex that unroll over a finger.

Safer Sex Chart

If you choose to go at it uncovered, here is what you are at risk for. Make an informed decision!

Unprotected Fellatio (Giving)

High Risk	Moderate Risk	No Risk	N/A
Gonorrhea	Chlamydia	Hepatitis A	Bacterial vaginosis
Hepatitis B	HIV	Hepatitis C	Vaginitis
Herpes	HPV		
Syphilis	Lice/scabies		

Unprotected Fellatio (Getting)

High Risk	Moderate Risk	No Risk	N/A
Gonorrhea	Chlamydia	Hepatitis A	Bacterial vaginosis
Herpes	Hepatitis B	Hepatitis C	Vaginitis
Syphilis	HIV		
	HPV		
	Lice/scabies		

Unprotected Cunnilingus (Giving)

High Risk	Moderate Risk	No Risk	N/A
Gonorrhea	HIV	Chlamydia	Bacterial vaginosis
Herpes	HPV	Hepatitis A	Vaginitis
Syphilis	Lice/scabies	Hepatitis B	
		Hepatitis C	

Unprotected Cunnilingus (Getting)

High Risk	Moderate Risk	No Risk	N/A
Gonorrhea	Chlamydia	Hepatitis A	Bacterial vaginosis
Herpes	HPV	Hepatitis B	Vaginitis
Syphilis	Lice/scabies	Hepatitis C	
		HIV	

Unprotected Rimming (Giving)

High Risk	Moderate Risk	No Risk	N/A
Gonorrhea	Chlamydia	None	Bacterial vaginosis
Hepatitis A	Hepatitis C		Vaginitis
Hepatitis B	HIV		
Herpes	Lice/scabies		
HPV			
Syphilis			

Unprotected Rimming (Getting)

High Risk	Moderate Risk	No Risk	N/A
Gonorrhea	Chlamydia	Hepatitis A	Bacterial vaginosis
Hepatitis B	Hepatitis C		Vaginitis
Herpes	HIV		
Syphilis	HPV		
	Lice/scabies		

Sharing Sex Toys

High Risk	Moderate Risk	No Risk	N/A
Chlamydia	Bacterial vaginosis	None	None
Gonorrhea	Hepatitis A		
Hepatitis B	Hepatitis C		
HIV	Herpes		
Syphilis	HPV		
	Lice/scabies		
	Vaginitis		

Dry Kissing

High Risk	Moderate Risk	No Risk	N/A
None	None	Bacterial vaginosis	None
		Chlamydia	
		Gonorrhea	
		Hepatitis A	
		Hepatitis B	
		Hepatitis C	
		Herpes	
		HIV	
		HPV	
		Lice/scabies	
		Syphilis	

Deep Kissing

High Risk	Moderate Risk	No Risk	N/A
None	Gonorrhea	Chlamydia	Bacterial vaginosis
	Hepatitis B	Hepatitis A	Vaginitis
	Herpes	Hepatitis C	
	HPV	HIV	
	Syphilis	Lice/scabies	

Ejaculation in Eyes

High Risk	Moderate Risk	No Risk	N/A
Chlamydia*	HIV	Hepatitis A	Bacterial vaginosis
Gonorrhea*	HPV	Hepatitis C	Lice/scabies
Hepatitis B			Vaginitis
Herpes			
Syphilis*			

* Chlamydia, gonorrhea, and syphilis can cause conjunctivitis.

Ejaculation on Exterior of Female Genitals

High Risk	Moderate Risk	No Risk	N/A
Gonorrhea	Chlamydia	None	Bacterial vaginosis
Hepatitis A	Hepatitis C		Lice/scabies
Hepatitis B	HIV		Vaginitis
Herpes			
HPV			
Syphilis			

Ejaculation in Nose

High Risk	Moderate Risk	No Risk	N/A
Chlamydia	HIV	None	Bacterial vaginosis
Gonorrhea	HPV		Hepatitis A
Hepatitis B			Hepatitis C
Herpes			Lice/scabies
Syphilis			Vaginitis

Anal to Oral Contact (Penis or Sex Toy)

High Risk	Moderate Risk	No Risk	N/A
Gonorrhea	Chlamydia	Lice/scabies	Bacterial vaginosis
Hepatitis A	Hepatitis C		Vaginitis
Hepatitis B	HIV		
Herpes			
HPV			
Syphilis			

Unprotected Anal/Vaginal Contact

High Risk	Moderate Risk	No Risk	N/A
Bacterial vaginosis	Hepatitis C	None	Lice/scabies
Chlamydia			
Gonorrhea			
Hepatitis A			
Hepatitis B			
Herpes			
HIV			
HPV			
Syphilis			

Unprotected Penis/Vagina Sex

High Risk	Moderate Risk	No Risk	N/A
Bacterial vaginosis	Hepatitis A	None	None
Chlamydia	Hepatitis C		
Gonorrhea			
Hepatitis B			
Herpes			
HIV			
HPV			
Lice/scabies			
Syphilis			

Unprotected Anal Sex

High Risk	Moderate Risk	No Risk	N/A
Gonorrhea	None	Bacterial vaginosis	None
Hepatitis B		Chlamydia	
Hepatitis C		Hepatitis A	
Herpes			
HIV			
HPV			
Lice/scabies			
Syphilis			

Resources

The listings below, organized by chapter, are intended to help you translate your fantasies into real-life sexual encounters. The list ends with mail order and retail outlets in the U.S., Canada, U.K., and Europe, where you can buy sex toys, safer sex supplies, and other accoutrements. And if you want to learn more about the explicit adult videos listed in each section, or simply about how to watch porn together, pick up a copy of my book *The Ultimate Guide to Adult Videos*.

Chapter 1:
Choose Your Own Adventure

Popular Fantasy Themes

BOOKS, EROTIC FICTION:

Sweet Life: Erotic Fantasies for Couples (1 and 2), and *Taboo*, Violet Blue

Naughty Stories from A to Z (1 and 2); *Down and Dirty; Bondage on a Budget; Naked Erotica*, Alison Tyler

Best Women's Erotica series, Marcy Sheiner

Aqua Erotica, Mary Anne Mohanraj

Wicked Words Black Lace Short Story Collection (series; 1–10), Kerri Sharp

BOOKS, NONFICTION:

For Yourself: The Fulfillment of Female Sexuality, Lonnie Barbach

WEBSITES, EROTIC FICTION:

Clean Sheets, www.cleansheets.com

Custom Erotica Source, www.customeroticasource.com

Nerve, www.nerve.com

Satin Slippers, www.satinslippers.com

When Fantasies Make You Feel Bad

BOOKS, NONFICTION:

The Erotic Mind, Jack Morin

The Survivor's Guide to Sex: How to Have an Empowering Sex Life After Childhood Sexual Abuse, Staci Haines

VIDEOS, INSTRUCTIONAL:

Healing Sex: Finding Pleasure and Intimacy After Surviving Sexual Abuse (S.I.R. Video)

Chapter 2:
Fantasies for One

A Tool for Men: The Squeeze Technique

BOOKS, NONFICTION:

> *The Multi-Orgasmic Man: Sexual Secrets Every Man Should Know,* Douglas Abrams and Mantak Chia

A Tool for Women: Your Vibrator

BOOKS, NONFICTION:

> *Tickle Your Fancy: A Woman's Guide to Sexual Self-Pleasure,* Sadie Allison

> *Sex For One: The Joy of Selfloving,* Betty Dodson

> *When the Earth Moves,* Mikaya Hart

The Golden Rules of Anal Masturbation

BOOKS, NONFICTION:

> *The Ultimate Guide to Anal Sex for Women,* Tristan Taormino

> *The Ultimate Guide to Anal Sex for Men,* Bill Brent

Chapter 3:
Fantasies for Two

Building a Fantasy Scenario

BOOKS, NONFICTION:

(For books on anal sex, see Chapter 2, above.)

The Bedside Kama Sutra: 23 Positions for Pleasure and Passion, Linda Sonntag

The Big Bang: Nerve's Guide to the New Sexual Universe, Emma Taylor and Loreli Sharkey

The Big O, Lou Paget

The Guide to Getting it On!, Paul Joannides

Hand in the Bush: The Fine Art of Vaginal Fisting, Deborah Addington

The Kama Sutra of Sexual Positions, Kenneth Ray Stubbs

Sex Toys 101: A Playfully Uninhibited Guide, Rachel Venning and Claire Cavanaugh

Toygasms: The Insider's Guide to Sex Toys and Techniques, Sadie Allison

The Ultimate Guide to Cunnilingus, Violet Blue

The Ultimate Guide to Fellatio, Violet Blue

The Ultimate Guide to Strap-On Sex, Karlyn Lotney

The Wild Guide to Sex and Loving, Siobahn Kelly

VIDEOS, INSTRUCTIONAL:

Better Oral Sex Techniques (Sinclair Intimacy Institute)

The Complete Guide to Sexual Positions (Sinclair Intimacy Institute)

Nina Hartley's Guides to: Anal Sex, Fellatio, Cunnilingus, Sex Toys (Adam and Eve Productions)

Toys for Better Sex (Sinclair Intimacy Institute)

The Ultimate Guide to Anal Sex for Women 1 (Evil Angel)

WEBSITES:

Freddy and Eddy, www.freddyandeddy.com

Tiny Nibbles, www.tinynibbles.com

Getting to Know Your Lover's Fantasies

BOOKS, NONFICTION:

365 Days of Sensational Sex, Lou Paget

Come Hither, Gloria Brame

For Each Other: Sharing Sexual Intimacy, Lonnie Barbach

Sex Talk: Uncensored Exercises for Exploring What Really Turns You On, Aline P. Zoldbrod and Lauren Dockett

Turn-Ons: Pleasing Yourself While You Please Your Lover, Lonnie Barbach

Chapter 4:
Role Play

Erotic Acting

BOOKS, NONFICTION:

Exhibitionism for the Shy: Show Off, Dress Up and Talk Hot,
Carol Queen

Sensuous Magic: A Guide to S/M for Adventurous Couples,
Patrick Califia

Where to Shop?

Look locally in costume shops, used clothing stores, and in
Halloween stores for inexpensive items. Sexy Halloween year-
round: www.sexycostumestore.com, naughty costumes at
www.trashy.com and www.pinupgirlclothing.com, plus-sized
fantasy clothing at www.ladybwear.com, and of course,
www.ebay.com. General information and inspiration can be
found at www.costumes.org. I've provided some links below to
sites that sell uniforms for professional use only. These sites are
for reference only: Impersonating police, firefighters, medical
professionals, and military personnel is against the law, and in
some cases, a federal offense. If you look authentic, please
keep it in the house, dungeon, playspace, or sex party.

Classic Roles

BOSS, CAT BURGLAR, CRIMINAL, DELIVERYMAN, ROCK STAR,
ACTOR, PIMP, SECRETARY, SLEAZY PHOTOGRAPHER, REPAIR-
MAN, SCHOOL AUTHORITY FIGURES, STRANGER, VICTIM:

Look in your own closet for appropriate clothing for these
characters; and shop for additional accessories to add realism.
Glasses make the boss or secretary, leather pants might make
you a rock star, fake gold chains and big rings can ease you into
pimpdom, and criminals are likely to wear ski masks and black

garments. You'll have to seek out specific repairman and deliveryman uniforms at used clothing shops or uniform stores.

BIKER:

You need leather. Or maybe some Pleather. Shop at a motorcycle store, a leather shop in your town, or online for chaps, vests, skirts, pants, or shorts. For authenticity, try these sites: www.stormyleather.com, www.mr-s-leather-fetters.com, www.chilhowee.net, www.harley-davidson.com.

CHEERLEADER:

www.cheerleading.net, http://cheerdeals.com, www.broadwayalbion.com

DOCTOR, NURSE, AND PATIENT:

For authenticity, www.anthonys-uniforms.com and www.allheart.com. Sexy: www.sirenssecrets.com/ naughtynurses.html, www.threewisheslingerie.com/nurse.asp. See "medical fetish" in the fetish resources below (listed under Chapter 9) for specialized gear (outside of stethoscopes and nurse's hats) sold for sexual purposes.

FIREFIGHTER:

The real deal is at www.fireoutuniform.com and www.chiefsupply.com.

FOOTBALL CAPTAIN:

www.bassco.com, www.teamsportswear.com, www.hitrunscore.com

HERO, HEROINE:

Your everyday clothes, of course. Maybe for underneath you'll want to check out www.costumecraze.com/Superheroes.html or www.superhero-costumes.com

HUMAN DOG, PONY, OR PET:

We're talkin' collars, bridles, leashes, human saddles. For the simple stuff, your local pet store or tack shop. For advanced, visit www.stormyleather.com, www.mr-s-leather-fetters.com, www.leatherdog.com (extensive links, including community resources for many types of animal play), www.the-stampede.org (ponyplay, extensive resources), www.equuseroticus.com.

MILITARY:

Army supply stores will have everything you need, cheap.

POLICE:

Can be thrown together easily—look around various websites for inspiration. The real thing is at www.cysuniforms.com, more at www.chiefsupply.com.

PRIEST, NUN:

Sexy and fun, a good selection is at www.costumecraze.com/Couples-Costumes.html. Real priest cassocks at www.zieglers.com.

SCHOOLGIRL OR -BOY:

Pretty much every stripper store, adult toy store, and costume shop has a risqué schoolgirl outfit, but sometimes the real thing is sexier. What you need is a plaid skirt, white top, and tie—or slacks and white top and tie, all found in your closet or local used clothing store. If you order the real thing online, as an adult you'll need to order children's plus sizes. Check out www.frenchtoast.com for inspiration.

Gender Play

Cross-dressing for sex is a blast. Men will don bras, panties, garters or pantyhose, skirts and dresses, heels (if you can find large sizes), and makeup. Look at www.cross-dress.com, www.tgforum.com, find oodles of links at www.lazycrossdresser.tv/links.html, and absolutely visit www.missvera.com. How-to books for male-to-female gender roles include *Miss Vera's Finishing School for Boys Who Want to be*

Girls and *Miss Vera's Cross Dress for Success,* by Miss Veronica Vera; *A Charm School for Sissy Maids,* by Mistress Loreli; and *The Lazy Crossdresser,* by Charles (Charlie Girl) Anders.

Women dressing as men will decide between boxers and briefs and slip into suits, workmen's uniforms, or any other masculine attire. Facial hair can be added with theater spirit gum and false hair (available at theater makeup stores), and you can strap on a dildo for form or function inside your pants. Get packing dildos and harnesses at www.goodvibes.com. Find further information, such as books and videos, in the fetish resources below (under Chapter 9). Books for female-to-male cross-dressing include *The Ultimate Guide to Strap-On Sex,* by Karlyn Lotney.

Age Play

Costuming for age play usually involves one partner being significantly younger, and that is where the focus of dress lies. Age play can be done with schoolgirl or -boy costumes, or taken further with adult diapers found at the adult baby resource www.dpf.com; more humorous adult baby mischief is at www.hubbies.com. Also check out www.foreverakid.com.

Chapter 5:
Threesomes, Foursomes, and Moresomes

BOOKS, NONFICTION:

The Ethical Slut: A Guide to Infinite Sexual Possibilities, Dossie Easton and Catherine A. Liszt

Polyamory: The New Love Without Limits, Deborah M. Anapol

Redefining Our Relationships: Guidelines for Responsible Open Relationships, Wendy-O Matik

Chapter 6:
Weaving a Spell: Striptease, Hot Talk, and Erotic Massage

BOOKS, NONFICTION:

Exhibitionism for the Shy: Show Off, Dress Up and Talk Hot, Carol Queen

How to Strip and Lap Dance 101

BOOKS, NONFICTION:

The Art of Exotic Dancing for Everyday Women, Leah Stauffer

Bedroom Games: Stripteases, Seductions and Other Surprises to Keep Your Partner Coming Back for More, Mary Taylor

VIDEOS, INSTRUCTIONAL:

The Art of Exotic Dancing for Everyday Women (Philadelphia Films)

The Art of Sensual Dance for Every Body (Self Appeal)

The Art of Dirty Talk

BOOKS, NONFICTION:

The Fine Art of Erotic Talk: How to Entice, Excite and Enchant Your Lover with Words, Bonnie Gabriel

VIDEOS, INSTRUCTIONAL:

Talk to Me Baby: A Lover's Guide to Dirty Talk and Role-Play (S.I.R. Productions)

Giving an Erotic Massage

BOOKS, NONFICTION:

Erotic Passions, Kenneth Ray Stubbs

Male Erotic Massage, Kenneth Ray Stubbs

Massage for Lovers, Tim Freke

VIDEOS, INSTRUCTIONAL:

The Best of Vulva Massage (The New School of Erotic Touch)

Fire in the Valley: An Intimate Guide to Female Genital Massage (The New School of Erotic Touch)

Fire on the Mountain: Male Genital Massage (The New School of Erotic Touch)

The Joy of Erotic Massage (The New School of Erotic Touch)

Chapter 7:
Strip Clubs, Phone Sex, and Call Girls—For Two

Phone Sex

BOOKS, NONFICTION:

Phone Sex: Aural Thrills and Oral Skills, Miranda Austin

WEBSITES:

www.phoneslutdiary.com, www.phonesexcentral.com, www.800phonesexsearch.com

Call Girls and Prostitutes

BOOKS, NONFICTION:

Paying for It, Greta Christina

Real Live Nude Girl: Chronicles of Sex-Positive Culture, Carol Queen

Turning Pro: A Guide to Sex Work for the Ambitious and the Intrigued, Magdalane Meretrix

WEBSITES:

Escort guides: www.epicdreams.com, www.eros-guide.com, www.janesguide.com

Legal brothels, Nevada: www.nvbrothels.net

Chapter 8:
Public Sex

BOOKS, NONFICTION:

A Guide to America's Sex Laws, Richard A. Posner and Katherine B. Silbaugh

WEBSITES:

Public indecency and "lewdness" laws by state: www.nudist-resorts.org/statutes.htm

Sodomy laws, international: www.sodomylaws.org/world/world.htm

Swinging

BOOKS, NONFICTION:

The Lifestyle: A Look at the Erotic Rites of Swingers, Terry Gould

VIDEOS, INSTRUCTIONAL:

Nina Hartley's Guide to Swinging (Adam & Eve)

Swinging: From Fantasy to Reality (Loving Sex/Alexander Institute)

MAGAZINES:

Loving More: http://lovemore.com

WEBSITES:

Instructional: www.sexuality.org/mgswing.html

World's largest swinging convention: http://Lifestyles-Convention.com

Lifestyle organization: www.PlayCouples.com

Network: www.theswinginglife.com, www.adultfriendfinder.com

North American Swing Club Association: www.nasca.com

Resources for swing parties in your area: www.eros-guide.com. Quality-rated and reviewed swing parties can be found at www.janesguide.com (site uses frames; look under Jane's Regional Guide: *your state or country*/Swinging).

San Francisco's Power Exchange: www.powerexchange.com

L.A. Couples and The Entertainium: www.lacouples.com

Alternative Sex Parties

WEBSITES:

www.eros-guide.com/events.htm

www.janesguide.com (site uses frames; look under Jane's Regional Guide: *your state or country* /Night Clubs/Resorts)

Chapter 9:
Fetishes

BOOKS, NONFICTION:

Come Hither: A Common Sense Guide, Gloria Brame

Sensuous Magic: A Guide to S/M for Adventurous Couples, Patrick Califia

Deviant Desires: Incredibly Strange Sex, Katharine Gates

Re/Search #12: Modern Primitives, V. Vale

Fakir Musafar: Spirit + Flesh, Fakir Musafar

BOOKS, EROTICA:

Best Fetish Erotica, Cara Bruce

MAGAZINES, FETISH FASHION (INCLUDING RUBBER):

Blue Blood, Demonia, Fetish Realm, Heavy Rubber, Marquis, Secret, Skin Two, Ritual, Taboo

WEBSITES, FETISH FASHION (INCLUDING RUBBER):

Blue Blood: www.blueblood.net

Dark Garden: www.darkgarden.net

Skin Two Magazine: www.skintwo.com

Secret Magazine: www.secretmag.com

Fetish Realm Magazine: www.fetish-realm.com

Marquis Magazine (German): www.marquis.de

Rubber and fetish fashion community network—check out the wide variety of fetish links in the "rubberdex" at: www.rubberist.net

House of Gord, the "home of ultra-bondage," is a shrine for extreme rubber fetishists and forniphiliacs (human rubberized furniture): www.houseofgord.com

Fetish parties: www.eros-guide.com/events.htm;
www.janesguide.com (site uses frames; look under Jane's
Regional Guide: *your state or country* /Night Clubs/Resorts)

San Francisco's Slick Fetish Ball: www.clubslick.com

WEBSITES, GENERAL:

Fetishes index: www.sexuality.org/fetish.html

For scores of links to thousands of individual fetish websites, visit
http://dir.yahoo.com/Business_and_Economy/Shopping_and_Se
rvices/Sex/Adult_Galleries/

Fewer sites, though less commerce-oriented than the index
above, are at http://dir.yahoo.com/Society_and_Culture/Sexuality/
Fetishes_and_Fantasies/

Personal pages on this index: http://dir.yahoo.com/
Society_and_Culture/Sexuality/Activities_and_Practices/

Index of fetish galleries:
http://directory.google.com/Top/Adult/Image_Galleries/

Jane's Guide has a reviewed fetish site section helpfully
organized by topic at www.janesguide.com; click on "Review
Index."

Chapter 10:
Erotic Dominance and Submission: S/M Fantasies

BOOKS, NONFICTION:

Come Hither: A Common Sense Guide to Kinky Sex, Gloria Brame

Different Loving: The World of Sexual Dominance and Submission, Gloria Brame, Jon Jacobs, Will Brame

Sensuous Magic: A Guide to S/M for Adventurous Couples, Patrick Califia

S/M 101: A Realistic Introduction, Jay Wiseman

BOOKS, EROTIC FICTION:

Best Bondage Erotica, Alison Tyler

Carrie's Story, Molly Weatherfield

Macho Sluts, Patrick Califia

Safe Word, Molly Weatherfield

VIDEOS, INSTRUCTIONAL:

Fetish FAQ (series, 1-4) (Ernest Greene and Mistress Ilsa Strix; Gwen Media)

Whipsmart: A Good Vibrations Guide to Beginning S/M for Couples (Sex Positive Productions)

Sweet Submission

BOOKS, NONFICTION:

Erotic Surrender: The Sensuous Joys of Female Submission, Claudia Varrin

The New Bottoming Book, Dossie Easton and Janet Hardy

When Being in Charge Turns You On

BOOKS, NONFICTION:

The Mistress Manual: The Good Girl's Guide to Female Dominance, Mistress Loreli

The New Topping Book, Dossie Easton and Janet Hardy

Captivity and Erotic Torment

BOOKS, NONFICTION:

The Erotic Bondage Handbook, Jay Wiseman

The Klutz Book of Knots, John Cassidy

The Seductive Art of Japanese Bondage, Fetish Diva Midori

Pleasurable Pain and Punishment

BOOKS, NONFICTION:

The Compleat Spanker, Lady Green

Family Jewels, Hardy Haberman

Flogging, Joseph Bean

Sensuous Magic: A Guide to S/M for Adventurous Couples, Patrick Califia

S/M 101: A Realistic Introduction, Jay Wiseman

Organizations and Private Clubs

The Exiles: woman to woman S/M: www.theexiles.org

QSM—Quality S/M books and nice link list: www.qualitysm.com

San Francisco's Society of Janus—site has extensive links to reputable regional organizations: www.soj.org

Seeing a Professional Dominatrix

HIGHLY RECOMMENDED PROFESSIONALS:

Cleo DuBois Academy of S/M Arts: www.cleodubois.com

Fetish Diva Midori and Fire Horse Productions—"Thoughtful erotic education for adventurous adults": www.fetishdiva.com

Mistress Morgana of San Francisco: www.mistressmorgana.com

Chapter 11:
Sex Games

Messy Fun

BOOKS, ART:

Messy Girls, Charles Gatewood

Aphrodisiac Seductions

BOOKS, NONFICTION:

InterCourses: An Aphrodisiac Cookbook, Martha Hopkins and Randall Lockridge

Temptations: Igniting the Pleasure and Power of Aphrodisiacs, Ellen and Michael Albertson

Make Your Own Porn

BOOKS, NONFICTION:

Erotic Home Videos: Create Your Own Adult Films, Anna Span

The Little Digital Video Book, Michael Rubin

Your Erotic Photo Shoot

BOOKS, NONFICTION:

The Little Digital Camera Book, Cynthia Baron and Daniel Peck

Photography for Perverts, Charles Gatewood

Webcams and Digital Images

BOOKS, NONFICTION:

The Little Web Cam Book, Elisabeth Parker

Chapter 13:
Safer Sex

CENTERS FOR DISEASE CONTROL

(AIDS and Sexually Transmitted Disease information)

1600 Clifton Rd., Atlanta, GA 30333

(800) 311-3435

www.cdc.gov

CETRA LATEX-FREE SUPPLIES

A product site for latex-free gear, catering mainly to the medical community (because so many medical professionals end up with latex allergies). Sells to individuals. Nice sitewide search.

(888) LATEX-NO; (510) 848-3345

www.latexfree.com

CONDOMANIA

Exhaustive site that sells virtually every condom under the sun, with fun facts, lots of condom information, and a helpful condom shopping guide.

(800) 9CONDOM; (800) 926-6366

www.condomania.com

GLYDE DAMS

Buy 'em here, by the dozen or in a party pack!

www.sheerglydedams.com

NATIONAL AIDS HOTLINE

(800) 342-2437

NATIONAL STD HOTLINE

(800) 227-8922

PLANNED PARENTHOOD

(800) 230-PLAN

www.ppfa.org

SAN FRANCISCO SEX INFORMATION

Sex information and referral switchboard providing free, anonymous, nonjudgmental, and accurate information about anything sex-related. Hours: 3 P.M. to 9 P.M. PST, Mon.–Fri. They also answer email questions.

(877) 472-7374; (415) 989-SFSI

www.sfsi.org

Resources for Sex Toys, Books, and Videos: U. S.

Adam and Eve

The retail face of the mainstream adult industry. Mail-order catalog and website of toys, books, videos, DVDs, safer-sex supplies, and lingerie, with a heterosexual focus.

P.O. Box 200, Carrboro, NC 27510
(800) 274-0333; (919) 644-1212
www.adameve.com

A Woman's Touch

Feminist sex store offering toys, books, and safer-sex supplies. Their website has great advice columns.

600 Williamson St., Madison, WI 53703
(608) 250-1928
www.a-womans-touch.com

Blowfish

Mail-order catalog and website of toys, books, videos, DVDs, safer-sex supplies, S/M gear, comics, and magazines. They feature individual reviews of their products and a strict privacy policy.

P.O. Box 411290, San Francisco, CA 94141
(800) 325-2569; (415) 252-4340
www.blowfish.com

Come Again Erotic Emporium

Woman-owned store with toys, books, videos, and lingerie; they also have a book and fetish catalog. Opened by Helen Wolf in 1981.

353 E. 53rd St., New York, NY 10022
(212) 308-9394
www.comeagainnyc.com

Eve's Garden

Woman-focused store and catalog of toys, books, and videos.

119 W. 57th St., Ste. #420, New York, NY 10019
(800) 848-3837; (212) 757-8651
www.evesgarden.com

Forbidden Fruit

Woman-owned and operated toy store/adult gift shop, fetish boutique, and body piercing/tattoo studio. A big supporter of the Austin S/M, fetish, safer-sex, and sex-positive communities.

www.forbiddenfruit.com

TOY STORE AND EDUCATION CENTER

512 Neches St., Austin, TX 78701
(512) 478-8358

FETISH BOUTIQUE

108 North Loop Blvd., Austin, TX 78751
(512) 453-8090

BODY ART SALON

513 E. Sixth St., Austin, TX 78701
(512) 476-4596

Good Vibrations

Mail-order catalog, website, and retail stores carry toys, books, videos, DVDs, safer-sex supplies, and comics. Promoting pleasure since 1977, Good Vibrations has a staff who are extensively trained and up-to-date on all things sex-related and are committed to dispensing accurate sex information about the products they sell. All products are individually selected and reviewed. The vibrators have volume and intensity ratings, and the website is loaded with sex information and a free magazine including articles and erotica. Mail order is open 7 A.M. to 7 P.M., PST. Carol Queen is their staff sexologist. Strict privacy policy.

(800) 289-8423; (415) 974-8980
www.goodvibes.com

> 603 Valencia St., San Francisco, CA
> (415) 974-8980

> 1620 Polk St., San Francisco, CA
> (415) 345-0400

> 2504 San Pablo Ave., Berkeley, CA
> (510) 841-8987

Grand Opening!

Retail store, website, and mail-order catalog of toys, books, safer-sex supplies, and videos; store has classes and events, some taught and hosted by owner Kim Airs. Great staff and terrific selection!

Mail order: (877) 731-2626
www.grandopening.com

> 318 Harvard St., Ste. 32, Arcade Bldg., Coolidge Corner, Brookline, MA 02446
> (617) 731-2626

> 8442 Santa Monica Blvd., West Hollywood, CA 90069
> (323) 848-6970

J.T.'s Stockroom

Gigantic online store with toys, books, videos, rubber items and lots of kinky toys, from beginner's to advanced. Great place to buy a Love Swing.

2140 Hyperion Ave., Los Angeles, CA 90027
(800) 755-TOYS; (323) 666-2121
www.stockroom.com

Pleasure Chest

Retail store, website, and catalog of novelties, toys, videos, and clothing. Super-friendly staff.

7733 Santa Monica Blvd., West Hollywood, CA 90046
(800) 75-DILDO; (323) 650-1022
www.thepleasurechest.com

Purple Passion

Retail store and website of toys, books, videos, magazines, and fetish clothing and shoes, plus a full selection of S/M and bondage toys and accoutrements. Mainly geared toward BDSM shoppers. Many of their BDSM toys are handmade by craftswomen, and impact toys are rated for intensity.

242 W. 16th St., New York, NY 10011
(212) 807-0486
www.purplepassion.com

Toys in Babeland

Website, retail stores, and catalog of toys, books, videos, and safer-sex supplies. Women-owned and operated, but open to all orientations. Strict privacy policy.

Mail order: (800) 658-9119
www.babeland.com

711 E. Pike St., Seattle, WA 98122
(206) 328-2914

94 Rivington St., New York, NY 10002
(212) 375-1701

Xandria Collection

Mail-order catalog and website of toys, books, videos, DVDs, leather, and lingerie. Betty Dodson is on their advisory board.

165 Valley Dr., Brisbane, CA 94005
(800) 242-2823; (415) 468-3812
www.xandria.com

Resources for Sex Toys, Books, and Videos: Canada

Come As You Are

No visit to Toronto is complete without visiting this community-oriented, worker-owned co-op retail store, with a mail-order catalog and website. They have toys, books, videos, safer-sex supplies, and educational resources, especially resources for the disabled. Products are handpicked and individually reviewed. Stores offer educational workshops. *Nous offrons des services limités en français.*

> 701 Queen St. W., Toronto, ON, M6J 1E6, Canada
> (416) 504-7934
> Mail order: (877) 858-3160
> www.comeasyouare.com

Good For Her

Woman-focused retail store carries toys, books, videos, and erotic art and hosts sex workshops, all geared toward female pleasure. In addition to regular hours, store has women-only hours.

> 171 Harbord St., Toronto, ON, M5S 1H5, Canada
> (416) 588-0900
> Mail order: (877) 588-0900
> www.goodforher.com

Lovecraft

Retail stores and website offering toys, books, videos, and lingerie. Possibly the oldest women-owned sex shop in North America— open since 1972.

Mail order: (877) 923-7331
www.lovecraftsexshop.com

27 Yorkville Ave., Toronto, ON, M4W 1L1, Canada
(416) 923-7331

2200 Dundas St., East Mississauga, ON, L4X 2V3, Canada
(905) 276-5772

Womyn's Ware

Retail store, website, and catalog of toys, books, and fetish gear, education- and woman-focused. Store hosts sex seminars.

896 Commercial Dr., Vancouver, BC, V5L 3Y5, Canada
Mail order: (888) 996-9273
www.womynsware.com

Resources for Sex Toys, Books, and Videos: International

Blissbox

A London-based website and mail order company that offers videos and DVDs, sex toys and accoutrements, and possibly one of the best adult video review databases around. The site is smooth, incredibly well designed, and easy on the eyes; provides fan information on porn stars and offers sex tips that are accurate and to the point. Videos and toys paired together are a perfect combination, and Blissbox knows it. The tone of the site is healthy, non-judgmental, supportive, and encouraging. It has a strict and simple privacy policy.

Telephone: (0845) 450-6655 (London, U.K.)
(Customer service 10 A.M. to 7 P.M. Mon.-Fri., U.K. time zone. Phone line is for orders only, with a £2 surcharge.)

Mail order: The website has a printable order form, though please check currency conversion rates if ordering outside the U.K.

Blackdog (their mail order company name)
P.O. Box 34984, London SW6 4XT, U.K.
www.blissbox.com

Coco de Mer

23 Monmouth St., Covent Garden, London WC2, U.K.
Telephone: (0207) 836-8882
www.coco-de-mer.co.uk

SH!

A women's sex shop.
22 Coronet St., London N1, U.K.
Telephone: (0171) 613-5458

Tiberius

Leather, Latex, and Tools.

Wien 7, Lindengass 2, Austria
Telephone: 43-1-522-040-74
www.tiberius.at

References

Addington, Deborah. *Hand in the Bush: The Fine Art of Vaginal Fisting*. Emeryville, Calif.: Greenery Press, 1998.

Albertson, Ellen, and Michael Albertson. *Temptations: Igniting the Pleasure and Power of Aphrodisiacs*. New York: Fireside, 2002.

Alexander, Priscilla, and Frédérique Delacoste. *Sex Work: Writings by Women in the Sex Industry*. San Francisco: Cleis Press, 1991.

Allison, Sadie. *Tickle Your Fancy: A Woman's Guide to Sexual Self-Pleasure*. San Francisco: Tickle Kitty Press, 2001.

Anapol, Deborah M. *Toygasms: The Insider's Guide to Sex Toys and Techniques*. San Francisco: Tickle Kitty Press, 2002.

———. *Polyamory: The New Love Without Limits: Secrets of Sustainable Intimate Relationships*. San Rafael, Calif.: Intinet Resource Center, 1997.

Anders, Charles. *The Lazy Crossdresser.* Emeryville, Calif.: Greenery Press, 2002.

Austin, Miranda. *Phone Sex, Aural Thrills, and Oral Skills.* Emeryville, Calif.: Greenery Press, 2002.

Barbach, Lonnie, Ph.D. *For Each Other: Sharing Sexual Intimacy.* Signet, 2001.

———. *For Yourself: The Fulfillment of Female Sexuality.* Signet, 2000.

———. *Turn-Ons: Pleasing Yourself While You Please Your Lover.* Plume, 1998.

Bechtel, Stefan, and Laurence Roy Stains. *Sex: A Man's Guide.* Emmaus, Penn.: Rodale Press, 1996.

Birch, Robert W. *Oral Caress: The Loving Guide to Exciting a Woman.* Howard, Ohio: PEC Publications, 1996.

Blue, Violet. *The Ultimate Guide to Adult Videos.* San Francisco: Cleis Press, 2003.

———. *The Ultimate Guide to Cunnilingus.* San Francisco: Cleis Press, 2002.

———. *The Ultimate Guide to Fellatio.* San Francisco: Cleis Press, 2002.

Brame, Gloria. *Come Hither: A Common Sense Guide to Kinky Sex.* New York: Fireside/Simon & Schuster, 2000.

———. *Different Loving: The World of Sexual Dominance and Submission.* Villard, 1996.

Brent, Bill. *The Ultimate Guide to Anal Sex for Men.* San Francisco: Cleis Press, 2001.

Bruce, Cara, and Lisa Motanarelli, Ph.D. *The First Year: Hepatitis C.* New York: Marlowe and Co., 2002.

Califia, Patrick. *Sensuous Magic: A Guide to S/M for Adventurous Couples.* San Francisco: Cleis Press, 2001.

Cavanaugh, Claire, and Rachel Venning. *Sex Toys 101: A Playfully Uninhibited Guide.* New York: Fireside, 2003.

Chia, Mantak, and Douglas Abrams Arava. *The Multi-Orgasmic Man: Sexual Secrets Every Man Should Know.* San Francisco: Harper San Francisco, 1997.

Chia, Mantak, Maneewan Chia, Douglas Abrams, and Rachel Carlton Abrams, M.D. *The Multi-Orgasmic Couple.* San Francisco: Harper San Francisco, 2000.

Daniels, Michael. *Woof! Perspectives Into the Erotic Care and Training of the Human Dog.* Las Vegas: The Nazca Plains Corporation, 2003.

Dockett, Lauren, and Aline P. Zoldbrod. *Sex Talk: Uncensored Exercises for Exploring What Really Turns You On.* Oakland: New Harbinger Publications, 2002.

Dodson, Betty, Ph.D. *Orgasms for Two: The Joy of Partner Sex.* Harmony Books, 2002.

———. *Sex For One: The Joy of Selfloving.* New York: Crown Publishing Group, 1996.

Easton, Dossie, and Janet W. Hardy. *The New Bottoming Book.* Emeryville, Calif.: Greenery Press, 2001.

———. *The New Topping Book.* Emeryville, Calif.: Greenery Press, 2003.

Easton, Dossie, and Catherine A. Liszt. *The Ethical Slut: A Guide to Infinite Sexual Possibilities.* Emeryville, Calif.: Greenery Press, 1998.

Freke, Tim. *Massage For Lovers.* Sterling, 1999.

Gabriel, Bonnie. *The Fine Art of Erotic Talk: How to Entice, Excite and Enchant Your Lover With Words.* Bantam, 1996.

Gach, Michael Reed, Ph.D. *Acupressure for Lovers.* Bantam Books/Bantam Doubleday Dell Publishing Group, 1997.

Gates, Katherine. *Deviant Desires: Incredibly Strange Sex.* San Francisco: Juno Books, 2000.

Gatewood, Charles. *Photography for Perverts.* Emeryville, Calif.: Greenery Press, 2003.

Gilbaugh, James H. Jr., M.D. *Men's Private Parts: An Owner's Manual.* New York: Crown Trade Paperbacks, 1993.

Gould, Terry. *The Lifestyle: A Look at the Erotic Rites of Swingers.* Richmond Hill, Ont: Firefly, 2000.

Haberman, Hardy. *Family Jewels: A Guide to Male Genital Play and Torment.* Emeryville, Calif.: Greenery Press, 2001.

Haines, Staci. *The Survivor's Guide to Sex.* San Francisco: Cleis Press, 1999.

Hart, Mikaya. *When the Earth Moves.* Celestial Arts, 1998.

Heiman, Julia, Ph.D., and Joseph LoPiccolo, Ph.D. *Becoming Orgasmic.* New York: Simon & Schuster, 1988.

Hopkins, Martha, and Randall Lockridge. *InterCourses: An Aphrodisiac Cookbook.* Memphis, Tenn.: Terrace Publishing, 1997, 2002.

Janus, S. S., and C. L. Janus. *The Janus Report on Sexual Behavior.* New York: Wiley, 1993.

Joannides, Paul. *The Guide to Getting It On!* Waldport, Ore.: Goofy Foot Press, 2000.

Kelly, Siobahn. *The Wild Guide to Sex and Loving.* Berkeley, Calif.: Ulysses Press, 2002.

Lotney, Karlyn. *The Ultimate Guide to Strap-On Sex.* San Francisco: Cleis Press, 2000.

Loreli, Mistress. *A Charm School for Sissy Maids.* Emeryville, Calif.: Greenery Press, 2000.

———. *The Mistress Manual: The Good Girl's Guide to Female Dominance.* Emeryville, Calif.: Greenery Press, 2000.

Masters, W. H., V. E. Johnson, and R. C. Kolodny. *Human Sexuality.* Boston: Little, Brown and Company, 1995.

———. *Masters and Johnson on Sex and Human Loving.* Boston: Little, Brown and Company, 1985.

Matik, Wendy-O. *Redefining Our Relationships: Guidelines for Responsible Open Relationships.* Regent Press, 2002.

Men's Fitness Magazine, with John and Beth Tomkiw. *Total Sex: Men's Fitness Magazine's Complete Guide to Everything Men Need to Know and Want to Know About Sex.* New York: Harper Perennial/Harper Collins, 1999.

Meretrix, Magdalene. *Turning Pro: A Guide to Sex Work for the Ambitious and the Intrigued.* Emeryville, Calif.: Greenery Press, 2001.

Midori. *The Seductive Art of Japanese Bondage.* Photographs by Craig Morey. Emeryville, Calif.: Greenery Press, 2001.

Morin, Jack, Ph.D. *The Erotic Mind.* New York: Harper Perennial/Harper Collins, 1995.

Paget, Lou. *The Big O: Orgasms, How to Have Them, Give Them, and Keep Them Coming.* New York: Broadway Books/Random House, 2001.

————. *How to Be a Great Lover: Girlfriend-to-Girlfriend Time-Tested Techniques That Will Blow His Mind.* New York: Broadway Books/Random House, 1999.

————. *365 Days of Sensational Sex: Tantalizing Tips and Techniques to Keep the Fires Burning All Year Long.* New York: Gotham, 2003.

Posner, Richard A., and Katherine B. Silbaugh. *A Guide to America's Sex Laws.* Chicago: University of Chicago Press, 1998.

Queen, Carol. *Exhibitionism for the Shy: Show Off, Dress Up and Talk Hot.* San Francisco: Down There Press, 1995.

————. *Real Live Nude Girl: Chronicles of Sex-Positive Culture.* San Francisco: Cleis Press, 1998, 2002.

Rodgers, Joann Ellison. *Sex: The Natural History of a Behavior.* New York: W. H. Freeman and Company, 2001.

Sonntag, Linda. *The Bedside Kama Sutra: 23 Positions for Pleasure and Passion.* Fair Winds Press, 2001.

Span, Anna. *Erotic Home Videos: Create Your Own Adult Films.* London: Carlton, 2003.

Stauffer, Leah. *The Art of Exotic Dancing for Everyday Women.* London: Carlton, 2003.

Stubbs, Kenneth Ray, Ph.D. *Erotic Passions.* Tucson, Ariz.: Secret Garden Publishing, 2000.

————. *Male Erotic Massage.* Tucson, Ariz.: Secret Garden Publishing, 1999.

Taormino, Tristan. *The Ultimate Guide to Anal Sex for Women.* San Francisco: Cleis Press, 1998.

Taylor, Emma, and Loreli Sharkey. *The Big Bang: Nerve's Guide to the New Sexual Universe.* New York: Plume, 2003.

Taylor, Mary. *Bedroom Games: Stripteases, Seductions and Other Surprises to Keep Your Partner Coming Back for More.* New York: Three Rivers Press, 2003.

Vale, V. *Re/Search #12: Modern Primitives.* San Francisco: ReSearch Publications, 1989.

Varrin, Claudia. *Erotic Surrender: The Sensuous Joys of Female Submission.* New York: Citadel Press, 2001.

Vera, Veronica. *Miss Vera's Cross Dress for Success.* New York: Random House, 2002.

———. *Miss Vera's Finishing School for Boys Who Want to be Girls.* New York: Doubleday, 1997.

Wiseman, Jay. *The Erotic Bondage Handbook.* Emeryville, Calif.: Greenery Press, 2000.

———. *S/M 101: A Realistic Introduction.* Emeryville, Calif.: Greenery Press, 1998.

ABOUT THE AUTHOR

VIOLET BLUE is senior copywriter at Good Vibrations, where she writes book and video reviews, which has her watching an awful lot of porn, and reading virtually everything imaginable about sex. She is a sex columnist and a sex educator. She is the editor of *Sweet Life: Erotic Fantasies for Couples, Sweet Life 2: Erotic Fantasies for Couples,* and *Taboo: Forbidden Fantasies for Couples,* and the author of *The Ultimate Guide to Fellatio, The Ultimate Guide to Cunnilingus,* and *The Ultimate Guide to Adult Videos.* Visit her website: www.tinynibbles.com.